Epidemiology
and
Health Policy

Michel A. Ibrahim
University of North Carolina at Chapel Hill

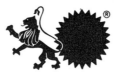

AN ASPEN PUBLICATION®
Aspen Systems Corporation

1985

Rockville, Maryland
Royal Tunbridge Wells

Library of Congress Cataloging in Publication Data

Ibrahim, Michel A., 1934 –
Epidemiology and health policy.

"An Aspen publication."
Includes bibliographies and index.
1. Epidemiology — Methodology. 2. Medical policy — Decision
making. 3. Health planning — Decision making. I. Title.
[DNLM: 1. Epidemiology. 2. Health Policy. WA 525 I14e]
RA652.4.I27   1985   362.1   85-3863
ISBN: 0-87189-100-X

Editorial Services: Martha Sasser

Library of Congress Catalog Card Number: 85-3863
ISBN: 0-87189-100-X

Printed in the United States of America

1 2 3 4 5

To

Betty, Daniel, Deborah,

David, and Peter

Table of Contents

Preface

What good may it do?
What harm may it do?
What harm may be done by not doing it?
Illingworth

In the face of unprecedented technological innovation and escalation of health care costs in a nation where chronic disease is prevalent and an aging population is increasing, health policies must be devised to govern the mammoth health care enterprise. The formulation of such policies must arise from a clear and well-accepted process but must also result in appropriate allocation of resources.

Resource allocation is largely determined by the principles of supply, demand, accessibility, and affordability, as well as the legislative and budgetary processes. The results of scientific research are yet to realize their full potential because research findings are often misunderstood or misinterpreted by policy makers. In guarding against inappropriate use of research findings, scientists compound the problem by introducing the assumptions and qualifications inherent in scientific inquiry.

Nevertheless, the weight of scientific evidence could provide powerful means for addressing the critical issues. The methods and tools of epidemiology offer an effective basis of a clear and acceptable process for setting health care policies.

In this volume the contributions of epidemiology to the study of health services and the formulation of health policies are presented. The method of investigation, gathering of information, data analysis, and interpretation of results are viewed with reference to general and specific issues in health policy. The primary focus throughout is the impact of a particular service or procedure on changes in health states of populations. A health service or procedure is considered one of many independent variables or determinants of the health state.

The book is divided into six parts. The first covers basic topics, including the derivation and use of health indices and disease classifications, the identification of sources of data for assessing community health needs, and the rules of evidence employed in the appraisal of causal relationships in epidemiologic studies. The second part is devoted to research design and analysis most appropriate for program planning and evaluation, such as time trends and ecologic correlations, cohort and case-control designs, before-after studies, and controlled trials. Policy issues of preventive services are illustrated in Part III with case examples of health promotion, disease prevention, and periodic health examination. Procedures and personnel are exemplified in Part IV by coronary artery bypass, computerized tomography, and the health care professional. In the fifth part, health care issues for the specific conditions of coronary heart disease, high blood pressure, and blood cholesterol are reviewed. Health care issues for selected segments of the population such as mothers, children, and the aged are presented in the final part.

The case examples presented were chosen to illustrate the value of epidemiology in formulating health policies. The philosophical, conceptual, and methodological underpinnings covered in this volume may be transferred and applied to other health service issues.

Acknowledgments

I was strolling in the exhibition area of the 1981 American Public Health Association meeting in Los Angeles when I was drawn to the books displayed in the Aspen Systems Corporation booth. There stood a low-keyed but determined and decisive young man. Mike Brown, director of publications, knew the publication business. We chatted about my course on epidemiology and its application to issues of health services and policy. He liked it and offered to publish a book on the subject. He has been most supportive and encouraging ever since.

Many thanks to the hundreds of students who took my course at the University of North Carolina at Chapel Hill and at the Epidemiology Summer Institute of the University of Minnesota in Minneapolis. Mention should also be made of the many teaching assistants, especially Frank Hielema. Their thoughtful evaluation and learned discussions have contributed immensely to the completion of this book.

Special thanks to Sally Zimney for preparing the graphic materials and to Dinah Lloyd and Jane Riley for typing the manuscript.

My deepest gratitude goes to the University of North Carolina, which is generously supported by the people of the state. I am extremely grateful to them for creating an academic environment where teaching and learning opportunities are abundant.

Part I

Epidemiologic Foundation of Health Services

Chapter 1

Epidemiologic Perspectives

During the last century doctors have affected such (disease) patterns no more profoundly than did priests during earlier times. Epidemics came and went, imprecated by both and untouched by either. They are not modified any more decisively by the rituals performed in medical clinics than by the exorcisms customary at religious shrines.

Ivan Illich

The publication of Ivan Illich's book *Medical Nemesis* in England in 1975 was received with mixed reactions. Some interpreted it as an attack on the medical care system, while others considered it thought-provoking and worthy of public discussion. His observation, however, draws attention to the importance of the evaluation of health or medical care programs and the role of such knowledge in the formulation of health policy.

Epidemics of plague in Europe, rickets in the United Kingdom, and pellegra in the United States reached their peaks and then declined. The fall of epidemics often occurs before the discovery of the appropriate treatment, as in the case of tuberculosis. Improvements in social and physical environmental factors and a better life style, dietary habits, and medical care play a major role in the decline of epidemics. The decline, since 1968, in mortality from cardiovascular diseases, particularly strokes and heart attacks, has been attributed to improved detection and treatment of hypertension in large segments of the population, improved diagnosis and intensive care treatment of heart attacks and strokes, improved dietary habits, and increased physical activity. The specific impact of each of these activities on the reduced mortality pattern cannot be determined, unfortunately.

The contribution of medical and public health practice to the well-being of the population can be assessed only if programs are evaluated appropriately before their implementation and large-scale utilization by the population. Otherwise the impact of specific medical and public health measures on the health state of populations may not be differentiated from that of other factors including "exorcisms customary at religious shrines."

The formulation of health policies has largely depended on two major concerns: first, economic and social, as in the case of Medicare (health coverage for the aged) and Medicaid (health coverage for the needy) and, second, political, as a result of the interests of pressure groups and major political figures, including presidents of the United States. Economic, social, and political concerns have impacted on health programs in a major but nonsystematic manner. For example, President John F. Kennedy's interest in mental retardation generated considerable funds for programs in maternal and child health in the early 1960s. President Lyndon B. Johnson's interest in heart disease, together with the civic worker Mary Lasker's political influence, resulted in the formation of the regional medical programs in the mid-1960s. These programs were designed to "conquer" heart disease, cancer, and stroke. President Gerald R. Ford, as well as his vice president, Nelson B. Rockefeller, developed interest in cancer especially after the discovery of breast cancer in their wives; that concern resulted in considerable public awareness as well as funds for cancer research. The pressures of interest groups, associations, and societies have likewise resulted in the establishment of research or service programs in areas of their respective interest.

Numerous medical procedures, advanced technologies, and intensive care units are introduced regularly. Their benefit either is not proven or cannot be proven since many already believe in their value; therefore proper testing by randomized trials is precluded. The American public, aided by powerful media coverage, has become fascinated by these advances and has acquired a set of values that inhibit raising critical questions.

Against this background it is not surprising that health policy is not based on answers to the right questions. Policy makers may search for answers to such fundamental questions about a procedure or program: "What good may it do? What harm may it do? What harm may be done by not doing it?" (Illingworth 1971, p. 254). Such answers may come from the special contribution of the science of epidemiology to the workings of health and medical services.

THE EPIDEMIOLOGIC APPROACH

Health planning and policy formulation in the ideal sense should apply to total communities and employ a centralized process, which facilitates an overview of the whole rather than selected health problems (Ibrahim 1983). This could become the third factor in the determination of health policy and would entail knowledge and understanding of the following:

- The distribution of deaths and diseases by demographic and social characteristics in the population. For this purpose, those who are interested in health policy may acquire a working knowledge in epidemiologic measures derived from vital records (for example, death and birth rates) and surveys (incidence and prevalence rates), health indices, and disease classifications that are pertinent to issues of health service. These measures may be used to estimate health *needs* (preventive and curative) of populations. Estimation of *demands* of the population may be undertaken through measures of health care utilization. Somewhere between the needs and demands may lie the kind of health services that could be offered to and possibly afforded by a particular community. Assessment of such needs and demands is a dynamic process requiring monitoring and surveillance. The state of health of the population could, therefore, be assessed periodically and become an integral component of the decision-making process.

- Assessment techniques of the impact of service programs on the health state of populations. Various steps should be undertaken to ensure that program evaluation produces meaningful data for policy makers. One must begin with an achievable and measurable *objective*, such as "to reduce the prevalence of uncorrected vision defects in school children." Policy makers depend on research findings to make programmatic decisions for initiating, maintaining, expanding, or deleting a particular activity. Therefore, results relevant to a decision should be predicted before the actual evaluation is begun. For example, a 50% reduction in the prevalence of uncorrected vision defects may be considered sufficient to warrant the continuation of the program.

  Services and procedures are designed to result in certain *changes* that in turn should produce an *outcome* or end result. Diet counseling as to the saturated fat content of food and the encouragement of the population to consume less fatty foods are procedures designed to produce a change—reduction in blood cholesterol levels—that in turn should result in reduced mortality from coronary heart disease. Program efforts, services, or procedures should not be used as substitutes for actual outcomes. For example, the establishment of 10 screening clinics where 1,000 school children are examined is a statement of effort and not an outcome.

- In an evaluation plan, a central question of whether the achievement of the desired objective can be attributed to the specific program. A satisfactory answer depends largely on the research methods employed. These methods range from the least rigorous observational type of investigations to the most rigorous experimental studies. Methods include analysis of time trends, ecological relations, before-after studies, case-control studies, cohort studies, and controlled clinical or community trials.

The epidemiologic approach to health policy differs from the approach of other sciences in that it provides for

- Defining the strategy of investigation, the type of variables, and the manner of data analysis and interpretation.
- Relating health problems and use of health care resources to defined populations, thereby identifying those groups who do not present themselves to medical care. Consequently health problems and health care provision may be viewed in terms of the entire population rather than only those who avail themselves to medical care (Cochrane 1972).
- Applying the knowledge of risk factors and the natural history of disease for the identification of its different stages. Early detection and prevention may thus become feasible.
- Developing a population-based health information system for health problems and their management (White 1976). The health information system is used to describe the population by demographic characteristics over time and across geographic areas. It is also used to describe the magnitude of, and changes in, health conditions of the population. Risk factors and subgroups at high risk in the population are identified. The system provides a description of health needs as perceived by health professionals, as determined by physical examinations, or as perceived by individuals on the basis of their responses to a health questionnaire. Surveillance and monitoring of health conditions and assessing the impact of health care measures on the entire population are important factors in organizing health services and allocating scarce resources.
- Focusing the impact of health care measures on the changes in the health state of the population. Within an epidemiologic context, a health or medical care program is viewed as one of the *independent* variables or determinants of health conditions of populations.

The last point is the most important distinguishing feature of the study of health services from an epidemiologic perspective. Concerns of medical care research and health policy analysis have largely been process oriented. That is, their focus has been on the efficiency of health services rather than the efficacy and effectiveness. The epidemiologic approach, with its primary concern on changes in health conditions of populations, adds an important element to the shaping of health policy. Considering health services as *another* factor in determining health states would place the provision of these services within their proper context: a means to an end rather than an end in itself (Figure 1–1).

The outlined formulation helps to clarify the other, and more traditional, use of epidemiology, which is concerned with the elucidation of causes of disease. The traditional use of epidemiology is based on the concept of agent, host, and environment interaction. The epidemiologist examines the relationship of personal characteristics and behaviors (such as age, gender, race, socioeconomic

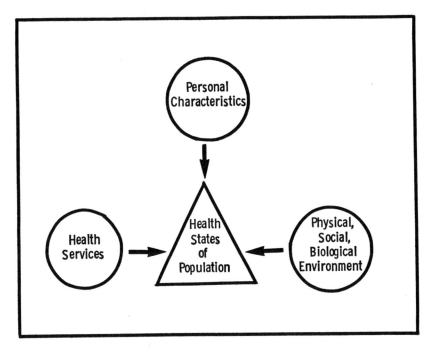

Figure 1–1 Determinants of Population Health States: The Etiologic and Health Service Uses of Epidemiology

status, smoking, and drinking) and environmental factors (such as water and air pollution, occupational toxins, and crowding) to health states of the population. In studying the etiology of disease, the traditional epidemiologist must take into account health service factors (such as use of a particular service) before making conclusions. Similarly the health service epidemiologist must take into account the personal characteristics and environmental factors before making conclusions about the impact of a particular service on health conditions of a population. In studying causes of disease or the workings of health services, then, the epidemiologist examines the interrelationships between a number of factors and a health state.

LIMITATIONS OF EPIDEMIOLOGY

Epidemiologists and health policy makers may take note of a number of issues that could interfere with an otherwise productive relationship. Epidemiology, like other disciplines, relies heavily on jargon, which is usually unfamiliar to non-epidemiologists. Good epidemiologic studies require a long time before meaningful results are obtained and are expensive. Unlike Great Britain, for example, we do not have an institutionalized health service system with definable populations. This problem coupled with geographic overlap in the provision of health services complicates the calculation of rates such as prevalence rates of a specific condition or utilization rates of a specific service. On the other hand health maintenance organizations (HMOs) with their defined populations, organized service delivery, and centralized and linked information system are excellent resources for epidemiologic studies.

Another limitation with the epidemiologic approach is the difficulty of isolating the effect of a health program from those of other factors. Changes in the health of populations may take years to emerge and are often due to many factors besides health programs. Political and administrative decisions are often made within a short time frame. Measures of effort (process) are more appealing than measures of impact (outcomes) because they are simpler and cheaper to collect and always produce positive results. In addition, administrators may resist collecting additional data for evaluative purposes because of their justifiable concern with unduly burdening practitioners.

In some instances epidemiologic studies cannot be designed to provide adequate answers to complex issues. Since scientific data are not the sole determinant of public policy, complex societal problems will have to be addressed "by political actions taken on our behalf by people who have the responsibility to make decisions based on ignorance" (Stallones 1982, 489). "A scientist may declare that the data are inadequate for decision making, but the policy maker has no such fence to straddle" (Stallones 1982, 490).

EPIDEMIOLOGY VERSUS OTHER DISCIPLINES

Several disciplines are useful in health services research and policy formulation. Each contributes in a specific way to decisions made in the health field (distinctive features of the various disciplines are presented in Table 1–1). There are similarities, differences, and overlaps among them. For example, the sources of data and methods employed by each of the disciplines are similar and include the use of patient records and observational and experimental study designs. Orientations and underlying theories or models differ, however. The orientation of clinical research is diagnostic and therapeutic; the orientation of medical care research is generally on processes of care. The underlying theory of clinical research is biologic, while the underlying theory in medical care research is behavioral. Epidemiologic research on the other hand is concerned with population health states and derives from biological, behavioral, and probabilistic theories and models.

Table 1–1 Distinctive Features of Disciplines Relevant to Health Services Research and Policy Making

Research	Orientation	Source of Data/Method	Theory/Model
Clinical	Diagnostic & therapeutic	Patient records/ observational & experimental	Biological
Medical care	Care processes	Patient records & surveys/ observational	Behavioral
Sociological	Human behavior	Surveys/observational	Behavioral
Demographic	Population dynamics	Registration & censuses/ observational	Biological/ probabilistic
Biostatistical	Quantitative	Patient records & surveys/ observational	Probabilistic/ mathematical
Operational	System analysis for decisions	Patient records & surveys/modeling	Probabilistic/ mathematical
Epidemiologic	Population health states	Patient records & surveys/ observational & experimental	Biological & behavioral/ probabilistic

HEALTH RESEARCH TERMS

These terms are commonly used in health service research and may be defined as follows (Sackett 1980).

Efficacy

Efficacy of a new health program may be defined as the benefit accrued above and beyond no program or a standard program. Efficacy is assessed by comparing the results in the group receiving the new program with those in the group receiving no or a standard program. The efficacy of an antihypertensive medication could be measured by the reduction in mortality and morbidity in individuals using the medication relative to the experience of individuals who are not using such medication. The virtual absence of poliomyelitis in those who are vaccinated reflects the degree of efficacy of the vaccine.

Effectiveness

Effectiveness of a health service relates to the acceptance and use of an efficacious service or procedure by those members of the population to whom the service is offered. The extent to which detection and treatment programs of high blood pressure that have been offered to various age-race-sex groups in a population have an impact on mortality and morbidity is a measure of effectiveness of high blood pressure control programs. The proportion of school children who are immunized against poliomyelitis is a measure of effectiveness of the intervention procedure.

Efficiency

Efficiency of an effective health service is measured by the extent of resources (financial and personnel) required to implement that service. For example, the extent of resources required to screen, and refer for treatment, the hypertensives in a population may be assessed for efficiency against encouraging primary care providers to check patients for high blood pressure levels.

Health care professionals and health policy makers have been concerned mostly with the efficiency of a service or procedure. Efficiency is important since it involves the use of scarce resources. However, if efficacy and effectiveness are documented first, programs found lacking in these measures would have been deleted, thus removing the necessity for raising the question of efficiency. Efficacy and effectiveness may be formulated and assessed with the aid of epidemiologic methods, and that is one reason why epidemiology may contribute in a meaningful way to the allocation of resources.

Investigators interested in health service research may also want to become familiar with the following terms (Starfield and Pless 1973).

Hawthorne Effect

The "tender loving care" received by subjects in an investigation may be the factor entirely or partially responsible for the favorable outcome observed in the group receiving the treatment and therefore may confound the real effect. In either case the benefits attributed to the intervention would be exaggerated. To help ameliorate the impact of this extraneous influence, another group of subjects— who are unaware of the study procedure while receiving the same intervention and on whom minimal data are collected—may be used for comparison if possible.

Placebo Effect

This effect may occur as a result of certain expectations by subjects whose condition would automatically improve due to the performance of the maneuver itself rather than its substance or content. The conditions of such people would improve as a result of swallowing an inert pill or simply going through the motions of a clinic procedure. Again, the impact of this effect may be reduced or eliminated by the inclusion of appropriate comparison groups.

Halo Effect

In this case a particular question or procedure may influence the nature of the responses to a subsequent question or procedure. For example, responses to attitudinal or behavioral questions may very well be influenced if they were preceded by questions on related knowledge. The halo effect may be remedied, at least in part, by randomizing questions or procedures whenever feasible.

CONCLUSION

The epidemiologic approach is useful in assessing community health needs and evaluating the impact of health programs and medical procedures. Focused on improvements in health states of populations as end results, epidemiology provides answers to fundamental questions about the beneficial or harmful effects resulting from a particular intervention. This knowledge, in addition to political and economic concerns, should form the basis of health policy making.

BIBLIOGRAPHY

Cochrane AL: *Effectiveness and Efficiency—Random Reflections on Health Services.* London, Nuffield Provisional Hospitals Trust, 1972.

Ibrahim MA: Epidemiology: Application to health services. *J Health Admin Ed* 1983; 1(1): 37–69.

Illich I: *Medical Nemesis.* London, Calder & Boyars, 1975.

Illingworth RS: Discussion of diagnostic examinations of the newborn by Norman T. Quinn. *Clin Ped* 1971; 10: 254.

Sackett DL: Evaluation of health services, in *Public Health and Preventive Medicine*, ed 4. John M. Last. New York, Appleton Century Crofts, 1980, pp 1800–1823.

Stallones RA: Epidemiology and public policy: pro- and anti-biotic. *American Journal of Epidemiology* 1982; 115(4): 485–49.

Starfield B, Pless IB: Research in ambulatory pediatrics. *Advances in Pediatrics* 1973; 20: 69–99.

White KL: Opportunities and needs for epidemiology and health statistics in the United States, in KL White, MM Henderson (eds): *Epidemiology as a Fundamental Science.* New York, Oxford University Press, 1976.

Chapter 2

Classifications and Indices

CLASSIFICATIONS

Continuous versus Discrete Characteristics

The development of a classification system or a health index requires the ability to differentiate the well from the ill, to determine the type and severity of illness, or to identify the cause of death. A condition that is defined as present or absent would fit the clinical model nicely, and its presence may be determined after specified criteria are met. Conditions such as angina pectoris or myocardial infarction are either present or absent on the basis of specified symptomatic, physical examination, or laboratory criteria. On the other hand conditions such as height, weight, or blood pressure may be expressed on a continuous scale of measurement and classified in several ways. Figure 2–1 is a schematic representation of these types of conditions.

Individuals possessing abnormal or indeed unusual values for a continuously distributed characteristic may be defined as those whose measurements are above or below two standard deviations. A second method is to divide the distribution into classes on the basis of subsequent mortality or morbidity experience. Blood pressure levels of 160 systolic and higher combined with 90 diastolic and higher would be classified as high blood pressure (or hypertension) on the basis of the increased mortality associated with these levels. A third way of classifying a continuous distribution would be on the basis of the unique experience of each class. For example, age may be divided into infancy, childhood, adolescence, adulthood, middle age, and aged. Each age class is associated with unique experiences that provide the justification for the classification. Finally, a particular

13

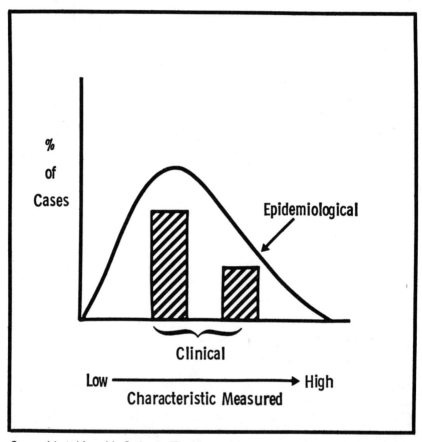

Source: Adapted from A.L. Cochrane, "The History of the Measurement of Ill Health," *International Journal of Epidemiology* 1 (1972): 89–92.

Figure 2–1 Schematic Representation of Categorical and Continuous Conditions

variable may be divided arbitrarily when a rationale for classification is absent. A variable may thus be classified into 5 to 10 units until the basis for a meaningful classification is found.

A distribution may be divided at a point where an intervention procedure would do more good than harm (Cochrane 1972). This concept of classification is particularly useful in health services research and health policy formulation. For example, a point on the distribution curve of hemoglobin values where iron treatment begins to have a favorable effect on health states would have important implications in the provision of health services. As attractive as it may seem, this approach is limited by its applicability only to treatable diseases and is somewhat impractical as it requires several randomized trials and is dependent on accurate definitions of good and harm. Nevertheless, it is an innovative concept of potential significance to health services research.

The Purpose of Classification

Nomenclature or *terminology* is a list of agreed terms used to construct a classification scheme. When applied uniformly, definitions and criteria enable the sorting of conditions into classes. The development of a classification system is the first step in any scientific inquiry whereby classified data facilitate statistical descriptions and inferences. William Farr, registrar general of England and Wales, stated in the sixteenth annual report, in 1856, that "any classification that brings together in groups diseases that have considerable affinity, or that are liable to be confounded with each other, is likely to facilitate the deduction of general principles" (International Classification of Diseases [ICD] 1967, p. xiii). Farr was also instrumental in developing the basic general arrangement, including the concept of anatomic site of the international classification of disease.

Classification may be defined as the orderly arrangement of data that serves a specific purpose. Over the years there has been an interest in developing a single classification system for universal usage, which would also promote comparability among studies. Such attempts have generally failed because conflicting requirements were inescapable in the pursuit of satisfying several purposes. Since most classification systems are developed for specific usages, attempts to construct a universal scheme are probably futile and may be abandoned.

Properties and Axes of Classifications

A classification scheme should ideally meet three properties:

1. Its classes must be mutually exclusive; that is, a case should be placed in one class only. When a case can be classified in more than one class, it should be placed in the class that would be most appropriate.
2. It should be exhaustive; that is, every case must be placed in a category. A miscellaneous category, not too large, may be developed to accommodate unusual or infrequent cases.
3. It should have a reasonable number of classes and a reasonable frequency of cases in each class. Ten classes would have been considered reasonable and manageable, but with the aid of computers the number of classes may be larger.

The axes of classification depend on the scientific purpose for which the classification schemes are being constructed. The physiologist, for example, would be interested in a classification that emphasized the systems of the body, the anatomist in organs of the body, the pathologist in the disease process, the clinician in causes of disease, and the third party payer in the length of the hospital stay. Axes of classification may be characterized as follows:

- Classification of a biologic measure such as blood pressure, serum cholesterol, blood sugar, and eye tension.
- Classification of cytological specimens as in the classification of cervical, breast, and lung cancers.
- Classification of diseases on etiology, anatomy, and function as done by physicians in clinical settings.
- Classification of diseases and deaths on the basis of etiology and anatomy as in the International Classification of Diseases (ICD).
- Classification of symptoms on the basis of patients' complaints during an office visit as in the National Ambulatory Medical Care Survey.
- Specialized classification schemes designed to describe conditions of selected populations. For example, the functional status of the elderly is classifiable on the basis of an Activity of Daily Living (ADL) scale of measurement. The Apgar classification is a specific system designed to describe the physical condition of the newborn.
- Classification of diseases according to health care utilization behavior as constructed for subscribers in the Kaiser-Permante Plan. For example, conditions are classified according to whether they require hospitalization.
- Classification that takes into account the length of the hospital stay for the purpose of reimbursement. The diagnosis-related group system (DRG) is an example.

The International Classification of Diseases, the symptom classification of the National Ambulatory Medical Care Survey, the Utilization Behavior Classification, and the classification of diagnosis-related groups deserve further mention.

Some Classification Systems

The International Classification of Diseases

The ICD is intended primarily for coding morbidity and mortality to obtain statistical summaries and analyses (ICD 1967). The ICDA refers to the International Classification of Diseases Adapted for Use in the United States. The adaptation is achieved by including a fourth digit to the conventional three-digit code of the ICD. Supplements to the ICDA are developed as the need arises to include classification of special hospital admissions, births, surgical operations, and operative procedures. Although the ICD cannot serve a universal purpose, it does provide a basis for other classification systems.

Although the ICD was designed initially to classify causes of death, the 1930 and subsequent revisions were expanded to include morbidity statistics. The sixth revision, developed after an international conference in Paris in 1948, was significant in that it symbolized the full international cooperation in the collection of health statistics and agreement on rules for selecting the underlying cause of death. It also combined morbidity and mortality classification schemes. Subsequent revisions included further refinements; the ninth revision of the ICD consists of 17 main sections on topics such as infective and parasitic diseases, neoplasms, and endocrine, nutritional, and metabolic disorders (ICD 1975). Each section is further classified to reflect the type and possible causes of the major group.

The National Ambulatory Medical Care Survey

In the National Ambulatory Medical Care Survey physicians are asked to record the patient's *principal complaint this visit* (Lawrence and McLemore 1983). Initiated in 1973, the survey provides continuous monitoring of ambulatory patients' visits to primary care physicians. The range of symptoms encountered in ambulatory care was grouped into 13 classes; each refers to a particular anatomic site and therefore conforms to the ICDA rubrics. For example, general aches, fever, fatigue, and exhaustion are classified under a general category; tremor, confusion, and giddiness are classified under nervous; acne and warts are classified under skin; pulse, murmur, and blood pressure are classified under cardiovascular. Periodic checkups and medical exams are placed in a last category of nonsymptomatic conditions.

The ambulatory medical care classification provides measures of the magnitude and nature of complaints by those who visit primary care physicians, as well as estimates of the volume of such visits on a national basis and by geographic and other factors. The system should prove useful in planning and evaluating health services, as in estimating the impact of a national health insurance scheme on health care utilization.

Classification by Utilization Behavior

The classification of conditions according to utilization behavior entails the grouping of diseases into classes most likely to result in similar medical care usage (Hurtado and Greenlick 1971). This system, consisting of ten classes, is constructed by grouping the conditions contained in the ICDA into a disease group and a nondisease group. The disease group is divided into seven classes of diseases: (1) generally requiring hospitalization, (2) diseases with high emotional component, (3) chronic diseases with no symptoms or nontreatable symptoms, (4) chronic diseases with treatable symptoms, (5) acute microorganism diseases, (6) acute nonmicroorganism diseases, and (7) undiagnosed diseases with symptoms. The nondisease category is divided into three classes: (8) pregnancy and complications, (9) trauma and adverse effects of external cause, and (10) nondiseases, refractive errors, or miscellaneous.

A second digit in the classification system provides further specificity. For example, diseases generally requiring hospitalization and requiring emergency surgery have a code of 11; those requiring surgery for malignancy, 14; acute microorganism disease produced by virus, 51, and by bacteria, 54; and prenatal and postnatal services for pregnancy, 81, and pregnancy complications, 82. Furthermore, the classification can be easily linked to the ICDA. For example, the pneumonias with classification code 13 correspond to the ICDA number 490–493.

The classification of conditions according to utilization behavior is useful in linking medical care usage to conditions. The amount of medical care resources required for the provision of services could thus be assessed. Analysis of utilization data over time might provide a clue about the potential impact of intervention measures in that visits for diagnosis and treatment of diseases would decrease while visits for preventive measures would increase.

Examination of utilization data by various age groups verifies the utility of the system. For example, 40% of the children under 4 years of age utilized services for acute microorganism diseases, and 36% utilized resources for preventive measures. Chronic diseases with treatable symptoms, acute microorganism diseases, pregnancy, and nondisease preventive measures each contributed 15 to 20% of health care usage in those 15 to 24 years old. Over half of those 75 years old have used services for chronic diseases with treatable symptoms, and 12% had diseases that required hospitalization (Hurtado and Greenlick 1971).

Diagnosis-Related Groups (DRG)

DRG is a classification system of hospitalized cases that has been used for reimbursing hospitals prospectively on a cost-per-case basis for the care of Medicare patients. In lieu of paying hospitals retrospectively according to expenses actually incurred, DRG is a move toward controlling the ever-escalating hospital costs by creating an incentive through reimbursement per case. The axis of this classification scheme is the length of stay. It was argued that ''if length of stay was defined as the dependent variable, one should be able to identify, in broad clinical categories, a relatively small number of independent variables that could be used to cluster cases into a manageable number of groups that were relatively homogeneous with respect to the dependent variable'' (Vladeck 1984, p. 577). Discharge diagnoses are coded according to the ICD and classified into 23 major diagnostic categories, such as diseases and disorders of the nervous system, diseases and disorders of the eye, and diseases and disorders of the respiratory system. Further subdivisions of each category are undertaken on such variables as surgical procedures, patient's age, and presence of complications in an effort to identify clusters of diagnoses that are homogeneous insofar as the length of stay within each cluster but different from length of stay in other clusters.

The sensitivity of the DRG classification system to severe cases characteristically placed in teaching hospitals was tested in a study in which patients treated in hospital-based facilities were compared to those treated in proprietary free-standing facilities (Plough et al. 1984). Severity groupings were determined on the basis of age, race, primary renal diagnosis, and accompanying conditions. The findings were suggestive that hospital-based facilities had a higher percentage of patients in the more severe groupings than did other facilities; if confirmed by other studies, this finding would have implications for reimbursement policies using the DRG classification.

The severity of illness was deemed important in developing a classification system that has an ultimate purpose of "case mix groupings that are homogeneous with respect to resource consumption" (Horn, Sharkey, and Bertram 1983). Six classification schemes including a severity of illness scheme and DRG were evaluated. The severity of illness system resulted in groups that were more homogeneous than those produced by other classification schemes. Homogeneity was judged by the degree of reduction in the variance of total charges for the use of tests and procedures for a number of specified conditions. Further developments and refinements of the classification systems for the prospective payment concept should provide a better basis for hospital reimbursement and may in fact result in the eventual containment of the rising hospital costs.

The prospective payment system will have a considerable implication on the practice of hospital care as well as out-of-hospital care. The role of hospital administrators, physicians, and others will change. The ultimate impact of this classification system on the health of patients remains unknown.

HEALTH INDICES

Process Measures

Health indices may be grouped into process, intermediate, and outcome measures. Examples of process measures include the number of physician visits, number of children immunized, and number of laboratory procedures and operations. These measures are important in medical care research, in medical audit, and in reference to the efficiency of providing health services. Process indices are acceptable as epidemiologic measures, if specified end results are known to follow the procedure. Since it is known that immunizations offer immunity against certain diseases, immunization rates of a community would be an acceptable proxy of outcome measures.

In medical care research, process measures in a particular practice are often compared with the aggregate experience of actual medical practice or with an ideal form of practice as determined by experts (Donabedian 1966). In either case, process measures are highly appropriate in evaluating clinical decision making of the new or expanded role for health professionals since this has been the traditional method of evaluating conventional health care providers. When analyzed thoughtfully, process measures could provide important information for the planning of certain health services. Although the volume of physician visits of a population may be of limited utility beyond administrative purposes, when examined by income levels and type and reason (diagnosis, treatment, or prevention) of visit, process measures bear added significance. For example, physician visits for preventive care are about three times as frequent in the higher economic groups as in the lower economic groups, but the latter generally make more visits for diagnosis and treatment than the higher economic groups.

Intermediate Measures

Intermediate measures reflect the immediate or short-range outcome of a care process. Examples include the number of asymptomatic unknown cases discovered by screening, adherence to medication and appointments, satisfaction with care, communication between health professionals and patients, and knowledge and attitudes about disease. Intermediate measures go beyond the process indicators since they relate to some sort of an outcome, albeit short-range. They are analagous to the process indicators in that their utility as epidemiologic measures depends on the assumption that desirable end results will ensue.

Outcome Measures

Outcome measures include those of disease, death, or disability (physical or emotional). These are truly epidemiologic measures in that they describe the health state of the population. The magnitude of a disease is measured by its incidence or prevalence. *Incidence* refers to new cases of a disease in a population in a defined period. Incidence is particularly useful in estimating the magnitude of acute conditions and other conditions of short duration. The proportion of the population affected by a condition (new and extant) at a given time represents a measure of prevalence. Prevalence is useful in quantifying the magnitude of chronic illnesses. Clues as to the relative effectiveness of a primary prevention or a treatment program may be obtained by studying the relationship between incidence and prevalence. The success of a primary prevention program would result in decreased incidence because of preventing new cases, while the success of a treatment program would result in decreased prevalence because of shortening the duration of illness.

Data on deaths are accessible and complete. Death rates, computed in different forms, are useful measures of the health of the community for diseases that are invariably fatal. The crude death rate is computed for all deaths of all causes in a population. Death rates may also be expressed for specific age, sex, or race groups. The weighted average of age-specific rates in a population forms a single age-adjusted rate for that population. Cause-specific death rates are obtained from the number of deaths attributed to a specific cause as listed on the death certificate. The validity of specific causes of death varies according to the condition, from 50% for coronary heart disease to 80% for cancer.

The case-fatality rate is the proportion of deaths from a specific disease or medical procedure in persons having the disease or exposed to the procedure. These indicators often serve as measures of quality of care. Case fatalities in teaching and nonteaching hospitals were compared for appendicitis, peptic ulcer, and hyperplasia of the prostate (Lee, Morrison, and Morris 1957). The rates were higher in nonteaching hospitals compared with teaching hospitals. This difference was most marked when the condition was severe, as in acute appendicitis with peritonitis, perforated peptic ulcer in 65-year-old and older males, or hyperplasia of the prostate in the 75-year-old and older (Figure 2–2).

Inferences about the quality of nonteaching hospitals should not be made in haste because patients admitted to those hospitals may be in poorer condition than those admitted to teaching hospitals. Furthermore, teaching hospitals may employ stricter criteria for patients whom they admit. If this were the case, patients in nonteaching hospitals would be expected to do worse than those in teaching hospitals. Analysis of data according to possible confounding factors such as age, sex, state of patient at admission, and complications did not, however, remove the difference in case-fatality rates between teaching and nonteaching hospitals. Furthermore, data collected on a subsequent occasion showed similar results.

Measures of disability or dysfunction may be obtained directly in the form of bed disability days, absenteeism from work or school, office visits, hospitalizations, etc. Questionnaires have been developed to estimate the health function of a community, which may be expressed on a continuum ranging from healthy to sick or from functional to dysfunctional. Such scales incorporate chronic conditions and symptoms of various diseases or simply measure functional status without regard to cause. The Cornell Medical Index has been useful in measuring emotional and general ill health (Abramson, Terespolsky, and Brook 1965). It consists of sections on symptoms referring to organ systems, fatigability, frequency of illness, diseases and habits, and mood and feelings.

A single index combining mortality and morbidity provides the means for comparing the changes in health states of a population over time (Sullivan 1971). The index is constructed with the aid of life table techniques in which life table

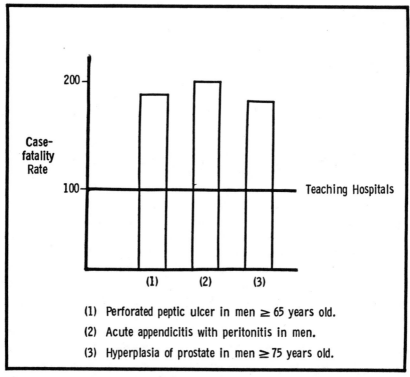

Source: Adapted from J.A.H. Lee, S.L. Morrison, and J.N. Morris, "Fatality from Three Common Surgical Conditions in Teaching and Non-teaching Hospitals," *Lancet,* October 19, 1957, pp. 785–790.

Figure 2–2 Case-Fatality Rates in Nonteaching Hospitals Relative to Teaching Hospitals

values are weighed according to time spent in disability by each age group. The result is an expectation of life free of disability. Total disability includes days of health care in long-term institutions, days when the person is unable to carry out major activities, and other days of restricted activity. The time an individual is expected to suffer disability of all forms over a lifetime is about five years.

The index provides useful information, as shown in Table 2–1. Although white and black men have a similar number of years remaining at age 65 (12.9 and 12.6), about three-quarters of the remaining years for white men will be spent free of disability compared with only 60% for black men. Corresponding percentages for white women and black women are 82% and 72%, respectively.

Table 2–1 Expected Years Remaining at Age 65, Total and Free of Disability, by Race and Sex Groups

(1) Race, Sex Group	(2) Expected Total Years Remaining at Age 65	(3) Expected Years Free of Disability at Age 65	(4) (3) as % of (2)
White men	12.9	9.5	74%
White women	16.3	13.3	82%
Black men	12.6	7.5	60%
Black women	15.5	11.2	72%

Source: Adapted from D.F. Sullivan, "A Single Index of Mortality and Morbidity," *HSMHA Reports* 1971; 86(4): 347–354.

Properties of Health Indices

A health index may be judged on a number of characteristics: reliability, validity, and prognostic value. Reliability refers to obtaining consistent results when the index is administered on two different occasions (test-retest reliability), when the index is administered by more than one interviewer (inter-interviewer reliability), or when the index is administered by an interviewer repeatedly to a group of people (intrainterviewer reliability). Indices should possess a high degree of reliability before they can be used for planning or evaluation purposes.

The validity of the index must also be assured before complete reliance is placed on the findings. Validity may be viewed in terms of face, biologic, or clinical validity (Sackett 1977). *Face validity* may be evaluated by direct examination of the items making up the index. These items should be precise, unambiguous, and acceptable as a convincing measure of the matter under investigation. *Biologic validity* is determined by the consistency of findings determined by the health index with our knowledge in human biology. For example, better physiological functions should be found in young people and in individuals free of disease. *Clinical validity* is estimated by the degree of agreement between the findings based on the health index and those on the basis of clinical assessment by a health professional. The clinical validity of an index is expressed by its sensitivity and specificity. The index sensitivity is its power to identify those individuals who truly have the condition. The specificity refers to the identification of those who truly do not have the condition. High levels (in the 90s) of sensitivity and specificity are desirable for a health index.

Another quality of an index validity may be termed *policy validity*. The health planner, administrator, and policy maker may be interested in this measure of validity. The question here is, When an index identifies a number of individuals with the condition (i.e., positive on index), what proportion of these individuals would be found to have the condition after being subjected to an elaborate battery of diagnostic tests? Similarly, when the index identifies individuals who are free of the condition (i.e., negative on index), what proportion of these individuals would be found to be free of the disease after the tests? For example, a 50% validity of a positive on index situation means that half of those found to have the disease on the basis of the index would have their condition confirmed after diagnostic tests. A 99% validity of a negative on index situation means that almost none of those individuals free of the disease by the index would subsequently be found to have the disease after the tests. These figures coupled with the information on the consequences of missing a positive case should aid in the allocation of resources, as in insurance payments for certain tests and procedures.

Finally, the prognostic value of an index may be evaluated in terms of its power to predict a defined outcome. The prognostic value may be best exemplified by the Coronary Prognostic Index developed by Norris and associates (Norris et al. 1969). The index is composed of six factors weighted according to their relative importance in predicting subsequent mortality from acute myocardial infarction in hospitalized patients. Each patient is given a score on the basis of the presence or absence of these factors. Grouped according to levels of these scores, patients with acute myocardial infarction experienced death rates that gradually increased from 3% in the group of patients with a low score to 78% in those with a high score. In addition to verifying the credibility of the index, this information provides a useful means for evaluating the impact of intensive care units on coronary heart disease mortality, as described in Chapter 12.

Whatever rigor is employed in its construction or in testing its properties, a health index may not entirely reflect the impact of health services. Sociodemographic factors may influence the magnitude of the index as much as or even more than do medical care services (Martini et al. 1977). Some outcome indices are sensitive to medical care programs, others are sensitive to sociodemographic characteristics, and still others are sensitive to both in different proportions. For example, the proportion of variation in total mortality may be explained more by sociodemographic characteristics than by medical care. The case-fatality rate within 48 hours for pneumonia is also explained more by sociodemographic factors than by medical care, while the case-fatality rate within 48 hours for cerebrovascular disease is explained more by medical care than by sociodemographic variables.

CONCLUSION

Classification schemes and health indices are required to determine the causes of morbidity and mortality, severity of illness, and outcome of programs or procedures in terms of population health states. The International Classification of Diseases is a key system of codifying morbidity and mortality and is often used as a reference for newly developed systems. Classification of conditions according to utilization of resources, such as hospitalization, is of special significance for health services research and health policy. The diagnosis-related groups classification has been developed to form a basis for the prospective payment system of hospitals.

Health indices may be grouped into process, intermediate, and outcome measures. A health index reflects the impact of medical services as well as changes in sociodemographic conditions.

BIBLIOGRAPHY

Abramson JH, Terespolsky L, Brook JG: Cornell Medical Index as a health measure in epidemiological studies. *Brit J Prev Soc Med* 1965; 19: 103–110.

Cochrane AL: The history of the measurement of ill health. *Int J Epid* 1972; 1(2): 89–92.

Donabedian A: Evaluating the quality of medical care. *Milbank Mem Fund Quart* 1966; 44(2): 166–203.

Horn SD, Sharkey PD, Bertram DA: Measuring severity of illness: Homogeneous case-mix groups. *Med Care* 1983; 21(1): 14–30.

Hurtado AV, Greenlick MR: Approaches and techniques—A disease classification system for analysis of medical care utilization. *Health Services Research* 1971; 6: 235–250.

International Classification of Diseases, Adapted for Use in the United States. Introduction (rev 8). US Dept of Health, Education, and Welfare, 1967, vol 1.

International Classification of Diseases, Adapted for Use in the United States. Introduction (rev 9). US Dept of Health, Education, and Welfare, 1975, vol 1.

Lawrence L, McLemore T: *1981 Summary, National Ambulatory Medical Care Survey,* Advance Data from Vital and Health Statistics, no. 88, US Dept of Health and Human Services, publication No. (PHS) 83–1250. Hyattsville, Md, National Center for Health Statistics, Public Health Service, March 16, 1983.

Lee JAH, Morrison SL, Morris JN: Fatality from three common surgical conditions in teaching and non-teaching hospitals. *Lancet* October 19, 1957, pp 785–790.

Martini CJM, Allen GJB, Davison J et al: Health indexes sensitive to medical care variation. *Int J Health Ser* 1977; 7(2): 293–309.

Norris RM, Brandt PWT, Lee AJ: A new coronary prognostic index. *Lancet* February 8, 1969, pp 274–279.

Plough AL, Salem SR, Schwartz M et al: Case mix in end-stage renal disease. Differences between patients in hospital-based and free-standing treatment facilities. *N Engl J Med* 1984; 310(22): 1432–1436.

Sackett DL, Chambers LW, MacPherson AS et al: The development and application of indices of health: General methods and a summary of results. *Am J Public Health* 1977; 67(5): 423–428.

Sullivan DF: A single index of mortality and morbidity. *HSMHA Health Reports* 1971; 86(4): 347–354.

Vladeck BC: Medicare hospital payment by diagnosis-related groups. *Ann Int Med* 1984; 100: 576–591.

Chapter 3

Data and Community Health Needs

This chapter covers selected national surveys; the leading health conditions in the United States; the estimation of the magnitude of a problem using published data; small area, or census tract data analysis; health needs and demands; and surveillance and monitoring of health states.

SELECTED SURVEYS

Among the important sources of data is the Health Interview Survey conducted by the National Center for Health Statistics (NCHS) on a national basis since 1957. It provides estimates of the incidence of acute conditions, prevalence of chronic conditions, disability days, and frequency of physician visits. The Health and Nutrition Examination Survey (HANES) was conducted by NCHS in 1971–74 and repeated in 1976–79; it included data on Hispanics in a special survey conducted in 1981. In addition to prevalence of chronic conditions, HANES provides estimates of the distribution of physiologic variables and assessments of the nutritional status of the population.

In the Hospital Discharge Survey, since 1964, more than 500 hospitals per year are surveyed by NCHS. Frequency of diagnoses and surgical procedures on discharged patients may be computed from the survey data. The PSRO (professional standard review organization) hospital discharge data are collected by the Health Care Financing Administration (HCFA) and are available on Medicaid and Medicare discharged patients since 1975. This is a resource for utilization statistics by diagnosis on patients in the PSRO system.

Data on visits to physician offices since 1973 are available from the National Ambulatory Medical Care Survey performed by NCHS. The volume and type of physician visits in the entire country or by region may be calculated from the data.

Analysis may be performed on patient symptoms (chief complaint) and diagnoses, as well as demographic characteristics of patients and specialty of physicians.

Vital statistics data on births and deaths by several medical and socio-demographic characteristics have been published regularly by NCHS since 1933. The National Death Index provides a unique resource for mortality data on a national basis. Cancer mortality surveys conducted by the National Cancer Institute give information on cancer deaths by county, type of cancer, etc. Monitoring and surveillance reports such as the Centers for Disease Control Morbidity and Mortality Weekly Reports (MMWR) are useful in estimating the magnitude and time trends of infectious diseases and other problems in the country.

A valuable resource may be found in the massive studies conducted by various national institutes of health. One notable example is the multisite collaborative studies conducted by the National Heart, Lung, and Blood Institute. The Multiple Risk Factor Intervention Trial (MRFIT) involved 20 research sites. Extensive data on about 300,000 men aged 35 to 57, examined initially in 1973–76, are available. The purpose of these trials was to find whether controlling the risk factors of high blood pressure, smoking, and saturated fats in diets would result in reduction in mortality. The Hypertension Detection and Follow-up Program (HDFP) involved 14 communities and was designed to estimate the effectiveness of antihypertension medication on the control of high blood pressure and reduction of mortality rates. Data are available on about 150,000 men and women aged 30 to 69. The Lipid Research Clinics (LRC) program included 12 research sites, with data on about 400,000 men aged 35 to 69, examined initially in 1973. The impact on mortality by reducing cholesterol by drugs or diet was the purpose of this large research project.

Finally, data from special surveys and studies conducted by individual investigators in selected areas may be accessible to health planners and policy makers. These resources are best identified through the general literature.

COMMON CONDITIONS

Community health needs may be assessed by the study of the prevalent conditions among its members. The conditions may be examined in various age stages from infancy to old age (National Center for Health Statistics 1982).

Health Conditions of Infants

Infant mortality has declined rapidly since the 1950s. The proportion of infants with low birth weight has also declined but at a slower rate. Furthermore, the rate of decline was slower for white infants than for black infants. The recent reductions in mortality have been attributed largely to neonatal intensive care, which is having its greatest impact on infants with low birth weights. Factors that influence infant mortality and low birth weight include maternal age, birth order, smoking, drinking alcohol or caffeinated products, education, nutrition, weight gain during pregnancy, prenatal care, and occupational and environmental factors.

The most striking difference in birth weight is between black and white infants. Black infants are about 2½ times as likely as white infants to be of very low birth weight (1,500 grams or less) and twice as likely to be of low birth weight (2,500 grams or less). Although this area requires further investigation, current knowledge of the risk factors affecting birth weight has not been fully translated into preventive health services.

Prenatal care is an all-encompassing method of intervention that could be used to motivate pregnant mothers to modify their behavior in addition to providing necessary medical care. High-quality prenatal care beginning early in pregnancy holds the greatest promise for promoting the health of the mother and the infant and for reducing the racial and socioeconomic disparities in birth weight. Yet nearly 80% of white mothers and only 60% of black mothers begin prenatal care in the first trimester of pregnancy. This situation is even worse for the most vulnerable, that is, teenage pregnant mothers and poorly educated mothers.

Another concern related to infants and mothers is the rising interest in home deliveries among many women, especially the more educated. The idea is attractive because of the minimal disruption to family life, the warmth and comfort of one's own home, and possible economic considerations. What might happen if this trend grows? What would be the implications for the mother's health and the infant's future? How would the system of medical or health care cope with this new demand? Who will do the deliveries: physicians, nurses, nurse midwives, or simply lay people who are especially trained for the task at hand? What would become of the licensure situation?

Health Conditions of Individuals Aged 1–14

The death rate in individuals aged 1–14 years has declined dramatically since the turn of the century. However, accidents have replaced the major diseases as important risks to this group. Accidents other than automobile make up better than half of the deaths due to all accidents. These include drowning, residential fires, and poisoning at home. The most important determining factor in this case is lack of appropriate supervision. Childproof packaging contributed immeasurably to the decline in poisoning. Important determinants of automobile accidents include dangerous driving and nonuse of seat belts or car safety restraints for babies. Wearing seat belts and developing safe driving habits are not yet fully appreciated.

Childhood cancers are still common in this age group and their causes continue to be elusive and not well understood.

Health Conditions of Those 15 to 24 Years Old

The 15- to 24-year-old group is subjected to major stresses and strains as they go through this critical period. It is tragic to note that the death rate in these individuals is higher in 1980 than 20 years earlier. This contrasts to a decline in death rates in all other age groups. The leading cause of death in this age group is automobile accidents. This is followed by accidents due to other causes. Homicide comes next (except the black population, in whom the homicide rate approaches the motor vehicle accident rate). Cancer and heart disease follow. These causes constitute a substantial proportion of deaths in this age group and represent directly or indirectly deaths and injuries due to violence, alcohol, or drug use. Driving at high speeds and driving under the influence of alcohol are major determinants of fatalities due to automobile accidents. Homicides and suicides are associated with alcohol or drugs, and may be enhanced by the ready availability of firearms.

It should further be noted that unwanted pregnancies and sexually transmitted diseases are important and prevalent conditions in this group.

Health Conditions of the 25 to 64 Year Olds

Heart disease, cancer, and stroke are the leading causes of death in this age group. Major well-known risk factors for heart disease include saturated fats and cholesterol intake, overweight, cigarette smoking, lack of physical activity, and stresses and strains of modern living. High blood pressure is an important risk factor for both heart disease and stroke.

Cancer is the second most common cause of death in this age group: cancer of the lung in men and cancer of the breast in women. Cancer of the colon is the second most common cause of death in men and women. Many of the causes of cancer are unknown or not understood. However, many risk factors have been identified, such as cigarette smoking, alcohol intake, certain diets, exposure to radiation, and other environmental and occupational factors.

Convincing evidence for occupational exposure to certain chemicals incriminates some 20 chemicals and compounds as major carcinogenic factors to humans. More than 2,300 other specific chemicals may be suspected as cancer-producing agents. Industrial and agricultural disposal of certain wastes have polluted entire communities and are posing considerable risks to human life. Many water supplies are contaminated with pesticides, bacteria, trihalomethanes, and other products. The carcinogenic potential of occupational and general environmental exposures may be enormous.

Health Conditions of the Elderly

The continued increase in absolute and relative terms of the elderly population (individuals 65 years old and older) is due to decreases in mortality coupled with decline in fertility. Therefore, the number of older persons and the proportion of older to younger persons have increased. This segment of the population increased to about 25 million and accounted for 11% of the population in 1980. A measure of dependency used by demographers is the ratio of the elderly population to the work force. This ratio has grown from 12% in 1940 to 20% in 1980. The sex composition of the elderly has also changed, in 1980 there were only 7 men to 10 women.

The three leading causes of death among the elderly continue to be heart disease, cancer, and stroke, which account for three of every four deaths in this population. Cardiovascular disease mortality has witnessed gradual decline since 1950 and some substantial decline since 1968. The decrease has averaged about 2% for men and about 3½% for women annually. Cancer death rates among the elderly have continued to rise since 1900. Cancer mortality has increased an average of 1% annually between 1950 and 1967 and 2% since. Most of the increase has been attributed to deaths from lung cancer.

In spite of the general decline in death rates among the elderly, major plights continue, including limited income, potential reduced access to medical care, sadness, depression, loneliness, and isolation. To keep the elderly healthy and independent represents both a problem and a challenge for policy makers.

THE MAGNITUDE OF A PROBLEM

Estimation of the magnitude of a problem using published data may be illustrated by the case of coronary heart disease as shown in the following steps:

- Define the population at risk for which the estimates are needed. In this example, the population at risk is men and women 30 years of age and older.
- Define the condition according to accepted criteria of diagnosis. Historical information and physical, electrocardiographic, and enzymatic findings are used to define the disease.
- Estimate the incidence of coronary heart disease in the population from published works. Age-sex specific incidence rates from "good" studies may be averaged to provide a best estimate. If the data are not available beyond certain age groups, extrapolation may be performed, if appropriate.
- Draw up the natural history or clinical course of the disease. For coronary heart disease, the clinical course may be described as deaths within one hour, deaths beyond one hour but less than one month, and deaths beyond one month but within the first year. From acceptable studies, age-sex specific case-fatality rates for each of these intervals may again be averaged to provide best estimates.

- Apply the estimated incidence and case-fatality rates to the respective population groups in the community for which the magnitude of the problem is to be assessed. The numbers obtained would provide estimates of magnitude of the condition at various stages of its course. To increase their precision, these estimates may initially be obtained for specific age, sex, socioeconomic, and geographic groups. These estimates may then be added up to give a total figure. The estimates of magnitudes are approximate figures with the advantage of being derived from published data without requiring costly surveys.

In the coronary heart disease example, average annual incidence rates per 1,000 population have been estimated from Framingham and other longitudinal studies (Ibrahim, Sackett, and Winkelstein 1969). These rates were plotted for men and women by age groups but extrapolated beyond age 50 because appropriate data were not available. These incidence figures were applied to the respective age-sex specific groups of a population at risk of 100,000,000. New cases of coronary heart disease on the order of magnitude of 700,000 men and 300,000 women were calculated.

Next, studies that examined the frequency of sudden deaths were reviewed. Definitions of sudden death varied in these studies from death occurring within a matter of minutes to death occurring within 48 hours. Reviewed for this purpose were studies performed on residents of Framingham, Massachusetts; civil servants of Los Angeles; employees of the Du Pont Company; enrollees in the health insurance plan of greater New York; males in Middlesex County, Connecticut; and employees of New York state, among others. Frequencies of sudden death in these studies ranged from 20% to 30%. For the present purpose, 25% was chosen as an estimate for deaths within one hour of the onset of coronary heart disease. Therefore, 250,000 sudden deaths would occur in the 1 million new cases of coronary heart disease in a population at risk of 100 million people (Figure 3–1).

Estimates of first-month case-fatality rates among patients with coronary heart disease were derived from appropriate studies and found to be in the range of 30% to 40%. A first-month case-fatality rate of 35% was therefore chosen. This rate included the 25% sudden death rate described previously, meaning that the death rate between one hour to one month was 10%, i.e., 100,000 deaths as seen in the figure. At the end of one month there would be 650,000 survivals and 350,000 deaths from the original 1 million new cases.

In a similar manner the best estimate for a first-year case-fatality rate was determined to be 40%. That is, 5% (40%–35%) for the period between one month to one year. At the end of one year there would be an additional 50,000 deaths, or a total of 400,000 deaths, leaving 600,000 survivals.

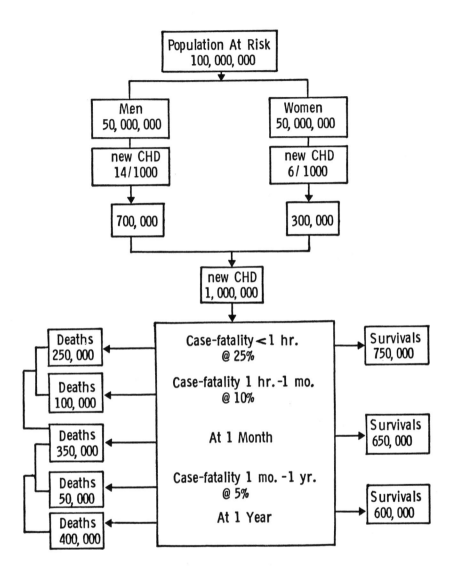

Source: Adapted from M.A. Ibrahim, D.L. Sackett, and W. Winkelstein, "Acute Myocardial Infarction: Magnitude of the Problem," in *Thrombosis* (Washington, D.C.: National Academy of Sciences, 1969), 106–116. Ed. Sol Sherry, Kenneth M. Brinkhous, Edward Genton, James M. Stengle.

Figure 3–1 Estimation of the Magnitude of Coronary Heart Disease in a Population of 100,000,000 Persons

CENSUS TRACT DATA

Census tracts could be grouped according to some health characteristic such as infant mortality into low, medium, and high (Figure 3–2). The same tracts could be grouped according to a socioeconomic index into low, medium, and high. Census tracts could of course be grouped into as many classes as desired or could be treated as units of separate tracts. Correlation analysis of the two indices (infant mortality and socioeconomic level) is performed to determine the degree of association between them. This way of analyzing data from defined geographic entities is termed *small area, census tract,* or *ecologic analysis.*

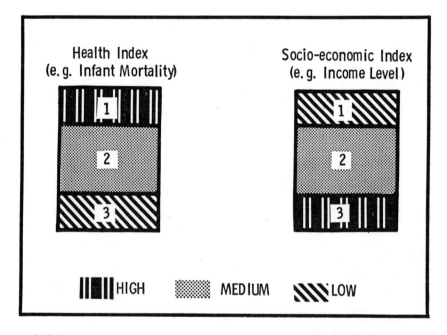

1, 2, 3 represent areas consisting of several census tracts each. The three areas are contained in a defined geographic entity such as a city. The city is classified on a health index in one instance and on a socio-economic index in another. Correlation analysis of the two indices may be performed.

Figure 3–2 Schematic Representation of Small Area or Census Tract Analysis

The method used for small area or census tract analysis may be illustrated by the works of Donabedian, Rosenfeld, and Southern (1965) and Anderson et al. (1965). Donabedian studied the association between socioeconomic characteristics of 90 census tracts in a wedge-shaped area of metropolitan Boston and the fetal and infant mortality occurring to mothers residing in those tracts. The analysis showed an inverse relationship between socioeconomic status and perinatal mortality rates. Census tracts with the lowest socioeconomic status had fivefold the perinatal mortality rate as those of the highest socioeconomic status.

The analysis of components of infant mortality provided important clues about standards of health care. The first-week deaths were predominant in census tracts with low infant mortality rates, as would be expected when high standards of health care prevail. This pattern was similar to the pattern of the United States at the time of the analysis (1950–54). On the other hand census tracts with high mortality rates exhibited patterns of infant mortality in which infant deaths between 28 days to 11 months predominate. This is similar to the pattern of infant mortality in the United States as a whole in 1915 as well as in partially developed countries. This analysis pinpointed areas of a modern American metropolis that appeared to be four decades behind national expectations.

Anderson et al. (1965) were able to identify geographic areas in Buffalo, New York, in need of maternal and child health services. At that time, President Kennedy's Panel on Mental Retardation concluded that "mental retardation and other disabilities were more frequent among groups receiving inadequate maternal and child health services." Therefore "it must be assumed that some of this morbidity can be prevented by the simple provision of maternal and child health services where they are needed" (p. 308). Census tract data and data from birth and death certificates were used to identify mothers and children at high risk. Indices of infant mortality, perinatal mortality, prematurity, birth weight, and obstetric complications of pregnancy were developed. Each tract was ranked on each of these characteristics. Tracts ranked high on three or more of these indices were considered at high risk and therefore in need of maternal and child health services. A circumscribed geographic segment designated as a core area was thus identified. Validation criteria such as percentage of children younger than 5 years old, percentage 65 years and older, and percentage of out-of-wedlock births were used to contrast the core area with the rest of Buffalo.

Once more the core area was verified to be at high risk as judged by the larger proportion of individuals younger than 5 years of age, the lesser proportion of individuals 65 years of age and older, and the considerably larger proportion of the percentage of out-of-wedlock births compared with the rest of the city. Further analysis within the core area showed subsegments that were at higher risk than other segments. This analysis may guide resource allocation, especially when resources are not sufficient to provide health services to the entire core area. Subsegments of highest risk may receive services before others within the high-risk core area itself.

DEMANDS AND NEEDS

It is important to distinguish between needs and health demands of a population. Needs are generally reflected by indices such as death rates, incidence and prevalence of acute and chronic conditions, and disabilities as determined by household or examination surveys of the entire community or a sample of it. Demands may be measured by the use of medical and health care resources and cannot be entirely indicative of population needs for health services. This is because of confounding factors such as the availability and accessibility of the resource and the socioeconomnic and education levels of the population served. Allocation of resources should ideally be made on the basis of health care needs rather than demands. Health care needs as determined by the prevalence of illnesses and magnitudes of mortality are generally associated positively with social indicators of the proportion of unskilled and unemployed in a community (Forster 1979). Health care resources as measured by general practitioner distributions in Great Britain were not associated with health care needs nor with social indicators. Social indicators such as the percentage of unskilled and percentage of unemployed may be useful parameters in the allocation of resources. This is especially so since they are relatively cheaper and more accessible than actual measures of health care needs.

SURVEILLANCE AND MONITORING

Surveillance is a French word introduced into English during the Napoleonic wars (Griffith 1976). It meant close watch over subversive activities and people in a community. *Health surveillance* may be defined as the continuous collection, analysis, and interpretation of data on individuals or groups to detect the occurrence of certain events and their putative causes for the purpose of control or prevention of diseases, evaluation of the impact of programs, and formulation of interventions (Foege, Hogan, and Newton 1976). Originally surveillance programs were concerned with infectious diseases when single individuals with an infectious disease were identified and isolated for treatment or monitoring of untoward effects of vaccination. Surveillance of infectious diseases is performed by the Centers for Disease Control and involves the examination of geographic and time trends of unusual occurrences for the purposes of control and prevention.

Generally surveillance requires three functions in this sequence: (1) data collection, (2) analysis and interpretation, and (3) decision making. The cycle repeats itself with additions or deletions in the data collection phase.

Surveillance may be performed using data from a variety of sources:

- Mortality data derived from death certificates and population censuses analyzed by census tract characteristics such as geographic regions and socioeconomic status of the population.

- Morbidity and disability derived from regularly available sources such as hospitals, industry, and schools. Morbidity and disability may also be obtained via surveys of representative samples of populations.

- Especially designed data source such as cancer registries, which combine mortality and morbidity and serve many surveillance uses. For example, time trends for site-specific cancers, cancer control measures, new treatments, and the emergence of rare cancers may be identified and evaluated using cancer registries.

- In addition to monitoring deaths, diseases, disabilities, and combinations thereof, biologic characteristics such as population growth, blood pressures, and nutritional status may also be the subject of surveillance (Irwig 1976). As an example, the growth of school children may be measured once a year and supplemented by additional information from students and parents on nutrition status, respiratory functions, etc. This method of surveillance allows the comparison of growth indicators such as height, weight, and skinfold thickness of equivalent age groups in successive calendar years as well as the comparison of annual growth rates of various age cohorts. The impact of nutritional intervention programs on the growth of children and the impact of environmental changes on the respiratory functions of children can be monitored effectively using this method of surveillance.

Surveillance may be used to effect changes in the practice of health care. The effect of surveillance on the number of hysterectomies performed unjustifiably in the province of Saskatchewan is an example (Dyck et al. 1977). Between 1964 and 1971 the number of hysterectomies performed needlessly increased 72% while the number of women older than 15 years of age had increased only 8%. A committee established a list of criteria by which the need for a hysterectomy could be retrospectively judged. A number of hospitals were reviewed, against these criteria, before and after the establishment of the committee. The average proportion of unjustified hysterectomies fell from 24% to 8% between the two reviews, or a reduction of 33% in such operations.

CONCLUSION

National surveys of health states give estimates of illness, disability, and frequency of physician visits and hospitalizations. Estimates of community health could also be derived from vital statistics on births and deaths. Leading causes of death differ among the various age groups as exemplified by deaths due to motor vehicle accidents in the 15 to 24 year olds and deaths due to heart disease, cancer, and stroke in the middle-age and older groups.

Methods are available for assessing community health problems from published information. Correlational analysis of census tract characteristics in relation to health conditions such as infant mortality could reveal geographic areas or population groups at high risk. Surveillance and monitoring of health states is an effective tool for documenting changes and trends that are useful in planning health services and inducing desirable changes in medical practice.

BIBLIOGRAPHY

Anderson UM, Jenss R, Mosher WE et al: High-risk groups—Definition and identification. *N Engl J Med* 1965; 273: 308–313.

Donabedian A, Rosenfeld LS, Southern EM: Infant mortality and socioeconomic status in a metropolitan community. *Public Health Reports* 1965; 80(12): 1083–1094.

Dyck FJ, Murphy FA, Murphy JK et al: Effect of surveillance on the number of hysterectomies in the province of Saskatchewan. *N Eng J Med* 1977; 296(23): 1326–1328.

Foege WH, Hogan RC, Newton LH: Surveillance projects for selected diseases. *Int J Epid* 1976; 5(1): 29–37.

Forster DP: The relationships between health needs, socioenvironmental indices, general practitioner resources and utilisation. *J. Chron Dis* 1979; 32: 333–337.

Griffith GW: Cancer surveillance with particular reference to the uses of mortality data. *Int J Epid* 1976; 5(1): 69–76.

Ibrahim MA, Sackett DL, Winkelstein W: Acute myocardial infarction: Magnitude of the problem, in *Thrombosis*. (Eds.) Sherry S, Brinkhous KM, Genton E, Stengle JM. Washington, DC, National Academy of Sciences, 1969, pp 106–116.

Irwig LM: Surveillance in developed countries with particular reference to child growth. *Int J Epid* 1976; 5(1): 57–61.

National Center for Health Statistics. *Health, United States, 1982*, US Dept of Health and Human Services publication No. (PHS) 83–1232. Public Health Service. Government Printing Office, December 1982.

Chapter 4

Rules of Evidence

Epidemiology is an investigative science concerned with the search for causes of disease, disability, or death through organized collection and analysis of data about the human population. Epidemiology is also an applied science concerned with the estimation of the magnitude of health problems in communities and the planning and evaluation of intervention programs with the ultimate outcome of improving health states of populations. Causes of disease may be found in the behavior of people, such as their dietary habits, cigarette smoking, or excessive drinking; in their biologic characteristics or constitutional makeup, such as high blood pressure or obesity; or in their environment, such as polluted air or water. Intervention programs may involve changes in human behaviors, environments, or provision of health services.

To identify the causes of a condition or the impact of a program on the health of the population, the epidemiologist depends on the knowledge and skills of several disciplines including social and biological, on a number of research methods and statistical techniques, and on a set of widely accepted scientific principles. The evaluation of the validity of the information obtained from epidemiologic studies requires the application of several "rules of evidence." Experience over the years has shown that application of these rules is crucial to the evaluation of cause-and-effect hypotheses. Inasmuch as the adherence to these rules of evidence before jumping to conclusions regarding cause and effect has been prudent, the same behavior may be observed regarding the formulation of a particular policy on intervention programs.

The following criteria—the range of studies, biases, and characteristics of association—are useful in assessing the design, data analysis, and interpretation of the findings of a given investigation or intervention.

THE RANGE OF EPIDEMIOLOGIC STUDIES

The persuasiveness of the evidence for linking cause and effect depends to a large extent on the research design employed in the investigation. Inferences about causality have been made on the basis of many types of investigations ranging from anecdotes and clinical hunches at one extreme to controlled experiments at the other. The two extremes form a continuum from the weakest method of studying a phenomenon to the strongest (Table 4–1).

At one end of the spectrum is the *experimental* design, where subjects or groups are randomly allocated either to the exposure of interest or to a control group. Experimental designs are often used to study causes of disease in animals. In

Table 4–1 The Continuum of Study Designs and Their Causal Implications

Study Designation		(1)	(2)	(3)	(4)	(5)	(6)	(7)	Inference
I.	Anecdotes	X			X				Speculative
	Clinical hunches	X			X				
	Case history	X			X				
II.	Time series	X			X		X	X	Suggestive
	Ecologic correlations	X			X		X	X	
	Cross-sectional	X			X		X	X	
III.	Case-control	X			X	X		X	Moderately suggestive
IV.	Before-after with controls	X	X			X		X	Highly
	Historical cohort	X	X			X		X	suggestive
V.	Prospective cohort	X	X			X		X	Moderately firm
VI.	Clinical randomized trials			X		X		X	Firm
	Community randomized trials			X		X		X	

(1) Observational
(2) Quasiexperimental
(3) Experimental
(4) Hypothesis generation
(5) Hypothesis testing
(6) Planning
(7) Evaluation

linking many diseases such as cancer, heart attacks, and stroke to their suspected causes in humans, experimental studies would be unethical as well as impractical. The benefits of a health program may be evaluated by clinical and community randomized trials. Such trials have been used to evaluate the impact of high blood pressure control programs and of the reduction of blood lipids by diets or medication. The causal implication derived from well-designed and executed clinical or community randomized trials is firm.

Epidemiologic evidence obtained directly from human population is generally based on *observational* rather than experimental studies. In such nonexperimental studies the investigator observes the phenomenon as it is occurring in nature and collects pertinent information to generate or test specific hypotheses. Unlike experimental studies, the characteristic opportunity for holding constant all factors other than the exposure of interest does not exist in observational studies. This basic distinction between the two modes of investigations makes it mandatory to adhere to the rules of evidence before conclusions are accepted.

Closest to the experimental studies along a continuum of research designs is the cornerstone of epidemiologic research, the *prospective cohort* study. In this design a population at risk is defined whose members have the potential of being exposed to the agent and could develop the disease. This population at risk is first examined to screen out persons with the disease. Individuals free of the disease are classified into those exposed and those not exposed to the agent. Both groups are followed prospectively to separate those who develop the disease from those who do not. The risk of developing the disease is calculated as the ratio of two rates: the rate of the disease among the exposed divided by the rate of the disease among the nonexposed. This ratio is called the *relative risk*.

Sometimes it is possible to reconstruct exposure data from records and perform the analysis as if the data were obtained in a prospective cohort study. The population need not be followed over time, resulting in considerable savings of time and money. This approach, the *historical cohort* study, is often used to determine if there is risk of disease in occupational settings. A variant of this approach, the *before-after* study, is used to determine the impact of a health program, for example, by comparing the case-fatality rate from heart attacks before and after the establishment of a coronary care unit. In this instance pertinent information is collected from records to reconstruct the various events.

In either approach a control group without the exposure or the health program must be included in the design to allow the derivation of meaningful inferences. The usefulness of this study design depends on the extent to which past exposure data are available, reliable, and valid. The difficulties in obtaining accurate, documented data place the historical cohort and the before-after studies farther away from the experimental study than the prospective cohort study on the continuum of research designs. In some instances the before-after studies are performed prospectively when the consequences of those exposed to the program and those not exposed are monitored, documented, and compared. This form of a before-after design is more of a variant of the prospective rather than the historical cohort study. It is not an experimental design because of the absence of randomization.

The next commonly employed research design on the continuum of epidemiologic investigations is the *case-control* study (Table 4–1). In the case-control study the frequency of exposure to an agent or utilization of a health service in cases who have the disease is compared with exposure or utilization in the noncases or controls who do not have the disease. In contrast to the cohort or experimental method, the investigator conducting the case-control study begins with the effect (or disease) and then looks backward in time for an exposure or service use that may be related to the effect. The relative risk or benefit cannot be determined directly in the case-control studies but can be approximated by what is termed the *odds ratio*, which is calculated from the proportions of exposure or service use in cases and controls.

Occasionally exposure information is classified in reference to an ecologic unit such as census tract, county, or city. These units may be categorized by characteristics such as urban versus rural, industrialized versus nonindustrialized, supplied by surface water versus supplied by ground water, or served by a community health center versus served by a group of private practitioners. Health states such as the infant mortality rate and proportion of individuals 65 years old and older may be computed for each ecologic unit. Relationships between certain characteristics and health states may be suggested after correlational analyses are undertaken. This type of *ecologic* study or small area analysis must be interpreted with caution and used only to generate hypotheses since the exposure information is so far removed from potential effects.

Time series and cross-sectional analysis may be included in this group. These observational studies are useful for planning and evaluating health services and generating hypotheses. The evidence produced by these studies is generally suggestive of a cause-and-effect relationship. The cross-sectional study involves the simultaneous collection of exposure and health states data on a sample of a population. Measures of associations between exposure and health states are easily computed. Time series analysis involves the examination of the fluctuations in rates of a condition over a long period in relation to the rise and fall of a possible causative agent.

Also at the weak end of the continuum are case-history studies in which investigators discover among a group of diseased individuals common exposure factors that appear to be more characteristic of the diseased persons than of the general population. Such case-history series provide a basis for generating cause-and-effect hypotheses, but because of their lack of any control group or rigorous information collection, causal inferences must be considered speculative until confirmed by more elaborate studies. At the far end of the spectrum from experimental studies are anecdotes and clinical hunches. Although speculative and usually based on highly selective information, anecdotes and clinical hunches do play an important role in hypothesis generation. In Table 4–1 the studies are listed in approximate hierarchical order ranging from those providing anecdotes to those providing experimental evidence. Some studies are designed primarily to generate hypotheses while others are designed to test hypotheses. Some studies are useful primarily for describing the community and planning purposes, while others are useful in evaluation of health programs. Of further importance is the causal implication of each study (assuming the study to be well conducted), which ranges from speculative to firm.

BIASES

Biases are sources of systematic errors that arise from faulty designs, poor data collection procedures, or inadequate analyses (Ibrahim and Spitzer 1979). These biases are inherently present in many observational studies but are of special significance in case-control studies. Biases may be categorized into selection, information, and confounding bias.

Selection bias results from a fault in the study design whereby certain individuals knowingly or unknowingly are selectively included or excluded from the case or control group. The systematic disproportionate frequency of the exposure variable in the cases or controls may result in a spurious measure of association. Epidemiologic investigations are laden with problems of selective bias. This class of bias includes selective admission, where cases of a certain disease are more likely to be admitted to a hospital; selective nonparticipation, where the refusal rate is high; selective survival in a study of survivors of a disease rather than of all patients; and selective detection, where diagnostic tests are made more often in the case than in the control group. Such systematic inclusions or exclusions of individuals in the case or control group could result in selection bias, which diminishes the validity of causal inferences.

The case-control study is especially susceptible to selection bias when subjects are systematically excluded from or included in the case or control group. Thus multiple control groups should be chosen instead of only one. When multiple control groups are used, at least one of the groups should come from the same source of care as the case group. Any selectivity associated with the cases would be expected to apply equally to that control group. A second control group may be chosen from the same neighborhood of the cases in order to control for socioeconomic differences or drawn as a random sample in order to achieve representativeness of the population.

Often overlooked by investigators, selection biases must be carefully avoided in the design stage of a study so that valid conclusions about the demonstrated associations may be made.

Information bias may result when the collected information on either the exposure variable or the health state is unreliable or invalid. Such information may result in the misclassification of certain subjects, which could produce a spuriously high or low estimate of effect. Historical data obtained by interviewing subjects without appropriate validation against recorded data are especially susceptible to one form of information bias termed *recall bias*. In an illustrative investigation of recall bias, it was found that 28% of mothers who had recent pregnancies resulting in fetal death or malformation reported drug exposures that could not be substantiated in either earlier prospective interviews or medical records (Sackett 1979). This is in contrast to only 20% of mothers with recent normal births who reported drug usage that could not be substantiated. That is, the former group were more likely to recall drug usage than the control group when the respondents' answers were compared to recorded data. Such a bias could have a profound effect on the results of a study that assumed that the data provided by the cases and controls were accurate.

Another example of the impact of information bias was shown in an investigation comparing reports of a family history of arthritis obtained from persons having arthritis against reports from their arthritis-free siblings. While 27% of the arthritis siblings reported that neither of their parents had arthritis, 50% of the arthritis-free siblings reported that neither parent had arthritis (Sackett 1979).

The consequences of information bias may be reduced by using only accurate recorded data, properly validating interview information, "blinding" the investigator as to the identity of the case or control, and adhering to an explicit and standardized method of data gathering.

Confounding bias may be defined as the mixing of the effects on the disease of the factors of interest with other (confounding) factors. The consequences could be either spuriously high or low measures of effect. Age, ethnicity, gender, and socioeconomic status are important confounders. This class of bias is widely recognized by most investigators, who attempt to minimize it in either the design or analysis stage of a study. In the design stage the consequences of confounding are alleviated by matching techniques and in the analysis stage, by stratification and multivariate analysis.

CHARACTERISTICS OF THE ASSOCIATION

Specificity of the association refers to the limitation of the relationship to "specific workers and to particular sites and types of disease and there is no association between the work and other modes of dying" (Hill 1965, p. 297).

Although an argument in favor of causation may be strengthened when specificity exists, specificity should not detract from the widely accepted notions that a disease or health state may be caused by more than one factor and that one factor may cause more than one disease.

The *strength* of the association increases the credibility of the findings, especially when the estimate of effect is several-fold in the exposed compared to the nonexposed group. In some cases the risk is obviously so great that the exposure factor is easily implicated. Death from cancer of the scrotum in chimney sweeps was 200 times greater than in other occupations, and cancer of the lung was 20 to 30 times as great in heavy cigarette smokers as in nonsmokers (Hill 1965). These observations leave little doubt as to the risks involved in sweeping chimneys or in smoking cigarettes. In many instances, however, associations derived from epidemiologic studies are of much lesser strength, and therefore causal implications are not readily apparent. Some guidelines for interpreting the strength of the association have been proposed (Daniels, Greenberg, and Ibrahim 1983). Considering that a relative risk value between 0.9 to 1.1 reflects no effect; 0 to 0.3 could imply strong benefit; 0.4 to 0.6, moderate benefit; and 0.7 to 0.8, weak benefit. On the hazard side, 1.2 to 1.6 could imply weak hazard; 1.7 to 2.9, moderate hazard; and ≥ 3.0, strong hazard.

A cause-and-effect hypothesis is further strengthened when the results of a study demonstrate that an *incremental* or *decremental change* in the exposure factor is accompanied by a corresponding change in the health state. Such results have been shown in studies where the death rate from lung cancer increased as the number of cigarettes smoked per day increased. The benefit of a health program may be shown to increase as the number or amount of services increases. Inferences about causal relationships between the factor or the program and the health state would be strengthened when these dose-response relationships are shown.

Consistency of the association with contemporary knowledge adds weight to the validity of the association. The association between rubella contracted during the first trimester of pregnancy and congenital cataracts in offspring was greatly enhanced by the biological determination that lens formation occurs early in pregnancy, when the lens is vulnerable to the harmful effects of rubella virus (Pitt 1957). On the other hand, when associations derived from epidemiologic studies conflict with other sources of knowledge, either biological or social, the validity of the association may be questioned.

Replication of the observed association is crucial in inferring cause and effect. Given the many biases that may affect any epidemiological study, it is important to ask whether the association has "been repeatedly observed by different persons, in different places, circumstances and times" (Hill 1965, p. 296). Only after studies have been replicated are epidemiologists willing to act. This is based on the assumption that it would be highly unlikely for all the biases in one study to appear in all the other studies.

The association between cigarette smoking and lung cancer has been repeatedly shown by numerous investigators, in different geographic areas and times, and by the case control as well as prospective methods of study. In reference to these studies, Bradford Hill (1965) remarked: "the same answer has been reached in quite a wide variety of situations and techniques. In other words, we can justifiably infer that the association is not due to some constant error or fallacy that permeates every inquiry" (p. 296). In the absence of replication, apparent associations must be interpreted with great caution.

These rules of evidence have been drawn from and applied to studies concerned with the elucidation of causes of disease. They may be applied just the same to health service research studies before their findings are used for making policies. The rules of evidence should serve as a guide for evaluating research findings.

Epidemiological studies need not satisfy all the criteria cited before an estimate of effect or a causal inference can be made—that would be both unwarranted and unrealistic. At the same time, to satisfy only a few criteria would be equally unacceptable. Epidemiologic studies must be subjected to critical and systematic appraisal and should be found to meet many of the rules of evidence before associations are considered persuasive and are used as a basis for policy formulation.

AN EXAMPLE

The application of the rules of evidence may be demonstrated in a large series of epidemiologic studies on the association between fluoridation of water supplies and dental caries. These studies contributed to the understanding of the relationship and guided health policies in reference to this matter.

The history of scientific inquiry into fluoridation of water supplies and protection against dental caries demonstrates the value of epidemiological studies when careful scrutiny is employed before conclusions are drawn. The issue of fluoridating water supplies has been debated in several communities for many years. Although a student of the political and behavioral sciences will find these debates rich in examples of community dynamics, the interest here is in the methodical fashion that characterized development of the scientific evidence.

As in many scientific breakthroughs, the initial relationship between fluoridated water and reduction of dental caries was discovered accidentally. At the turn of the century, Frederick C. McKay, a dentist in Colorado Springs, wanted to find the cause of a brown stain on the teeth of many residents. Eventually, through observations and experiments but especially after the chemical analysis of the water, excessive fluoride content was established as the responsible agent. It was also noted in Colorado and in several other states that the inhabitants of geographic areas supplied by water containing high concentrations of fluoride not only had stained teeth but also were free of caries.

Two studies were undertaken shortly after the inverse relationship between fluoride content of the water and dental caries was reported. One study included 2,832 children in 8 suburban Chicago communities; the second included 4,425 children in 13 other cities (Dean, Arnold, and Elvove 1942). Remarkable differences in the frequency of dental caries were noted between areas with water supplies containing less than 0.5 part per million of fluoride and areas containing higher amounts. Furthermore, dental caries were consistently lower (without a single exception) in every city where the fluoride content was high than in other cities where it was low.

These studies were published in the early 1940s, but research continued. In 1942, 316 children of Japanese ancestry were transferred with their parents to two centers—120 children to a center in California and 196 to a center in Arizona (Klein 1945). While the children in the California center consumed fluoride-free water coming from melted snow on a mountain, the children in the Arizona center consumed deep well water that contained 3 parts per million fluoride.

The two groups underwent dental examinations in the summer of 1943 and again in the summer of 1945. The dental caries experiences in 1943 were quite similar in both groups: 13.4 and 12.8 caries-free teeth for boys, 14.7 and 14.1 for girls. But after two years' residence in the designated centers, the number of teeth affected with caries per 100 teeth unaffected was twice as high in boys and girls residing in the flouride-free area as in those residing in the fluoride area. Further, the beneficial effect of fluoridation was most evident in the previously noncarious erupted permanent teeth of younger children (8 to 10 years old) than in those of older children.

Although the evidence accumulated by the mid-1940s was persuasive and sufficient for consideration of the question of preventing dental caries by artificial fluoridation, nevertheless, before proceeding in that direction,

> it was necessary to demonstrate (1) that fluoride at a concentration approximating 1 part per million in the water supply was safe and (2) that added fluoride did in fact produce the dental benefits associated with natural fluoride in the endemic fluoride areas. Only when this last attempt had been made could it be said with assurance that fluoride caused, and was not merely associated with, low caries. Trials of water fluoridation thus became necessary. (Dunning 1970, p. 372)

Several fluoridation studies were thus begun in 1945. In five years "it became so apparent that the trial cities would duplicate the experience seen in cities of similar natural fluoride concentration, the U.S. Public Health Service gave its endorsement" to communities wishing to fluoridate their water supply (Dunning 1970, p. 382). Reduction in dental caries of about 50% was commonly seen. Maximum benefits were again noted in the younger age groups whose teeth would have been mostly formed during the period of exposure to the fluoride.

Finally, the question of possible side effects of fluoridation was raised. This was of special concern since "an increase in the death rate among cancer-susceptible laboratory animals exposed to high-fluoride waters" was noted (Dunning 1970, p. 377). Several studies conducted in response to this important issue agreed "in showing no abnormalities, pathologic effects, or mortality changes that can be related to fluoride in the drinking water" (Dunning 1970, p. 377). The death rates from five causes, including cancer, were similar in fluoride and nonfluoride cities for the period 1940–50.

The fluoridation/caries example reveals that epidemiologic investigations constitute a powerful approach in establishing causation when several of the rules of evidence described previously have been met. The observation that more reduction in dental caries was found in younger children than in older children, confirming that longer exposure to fluoride of the newly formed teeth would result in maximum benefit, was consistent with prevailing scientific theories and knowledge. Cohort studies reduced the opportunities that could have resulted in selection bias. In addition to increasing confidence in the safety of fluoridation, the lack of association between fluoridation and several causes of death signified a degree of specificity of the correlation between fluoride and dental caries. The impact of information and confounding biases on the results was diminished by the careful and objective dental examinations and by the employment of stratification and various adjustments in data analysis. Finally, studies of different designs, conducted by different investigators in different geographic areas and at different times, revealed consistent findings—replication in its fullest form.

CONCLUSION

Scientists have agreed on a set of criteria—rules of evidence—that must be met before a conclusion about cause and effect is made. The persuasiveness of the evidence for linking cause to effect depends to a large extent on the research design. On one end of the continuum is the experimental design, which results in firm evidence, and on the other end are the anecdotes and clinical hunches whose evidence is speculative.

Biases must be searched for and eliminated in the design phase of a study or taken into account in data analysis and presentation of findings. Information, selection, and confounding are the most common biases.

The third set of criteria used in judging cause-and-effect relationships characterizes the association between an exposure and a health state. This set includes specificity, strength, dose-response, consistency, and replication.

The rules of evidence should serve as a guide for evaluating research findings. Epidemiologic studies must undergo systemic appraisal before their findings are accepted.

BIBLIOGRAPHY

Daniels SR, Greenberg RS, Ibrahim MA: Etiologic research in pediatric epidemiology. *J Pediatrics* 1983; 102(4): 494–504.

Dean HT, Arnold FA Jr, Elvove E: Domestic water and dental caries. *Pub Health Rep* 1942; 57(32): 1155–1179.

Dunning JM: *Principles of Dental Public Health Practice,* ed 2. Cambridge, Mass, Harvard University Press, 1970, pp 367–386.

Hill AB: The environment and disease: Association or causation. *Proc Royal Soc Med* 1965; 58: 295–300.

Ibrahim MA, Spitzer WO: The case-control study: The problem and the prospect. *J Chron Dis* 1979; 32: 139–144.

Klein H: Dental caries experience in relocated children exposed to water containing fluorine. *Pub Health Rep* 1945; 60: 1462–1467.

Pitt DB: Congenital malformations and maternal rubella. *Med J Austral* 1957; 1: 233–239.

Sackett DL: Bias in analytic research. *J Chron Dis* 1979; 32: 51–63.

Part II

Research Design and Analysis

Chapter 5

Time Trends, Ecologic Correlation, and Modeling

TIME TRENDS AND ECOLOGIC ANALYSIS

Reference has already been made to time series and ecologic studies in Chapter 3. In time series studies a phenomenon is described and analyzed over time. Ecologic studies refer to the description and analysis of health states by the characteristics of ecologic units. Ecologic units such as counties, states, or census tracts are grouped according to characteristics such as level of economic status or degree of urbanity. Mortality or morbidity rates or other measures of health states are contrasted among such groups. Time series and ecologic studies are useful in estimating community health needs for planning purposes and in judging the potential impact of intervention programs.

If there is a decline over time in mortality or morbidity rates of a condition, it is difficult to attribute the decline to a specific intervention measure. Many diseases escalated to epidemic proportions only to show steady decline thereafter. The reasons for such declines are often not entirely understood. Epidemic waves throughout the centuries have been exemplified by rickets in the United Kingdom and pellagra in the United States, which achieved epidemic proportions in the 1800s. As these deficiency conditions declined, they were replaced by infectious diseases that peaked in the 1900s. As infectious diseases began their decline, chronic diseases began their rise to peaks in the 1950s. Chronic diseases, especially coronary heart disease, stroke, and hypertension, have shown gradual decline early in the second half of the twentieth century, and they seem to be replaced by conditions of mental and social disorders and those resulting from acts of violence. These may peak early in the twenty-first century.

Factors other than the specific intervention, such as changes in the economic and employment situations, changes in the demographic characteristics of the population, or changes in behaviors or life style, may have resulted in the decline of the rates or at least confounded the impact of specific intervention measures.

Examination of time trends poses another problem, which relates to a phenomenon called *regression toward the mean*. It is likely that populations selected for participation in an intervention program are generally experiencing a more severe level of the condition than populations not selected. It is expected, therefore, that the health state of the population selected will show some improvements, at least early in the program, that are not necessarily due to the intervention procedure. These initial improvements may be due to regression toward the mean.

Gillings (1981) and others proposed a segmented regression method to test the impact on mortality of a specific program in a study region compared with a control region. The method does not require the collection of primary data but uses available data from birth and death certificates. The impact of the regionalized perinatal care programs on reducing perinatal mortality and decreasing differences among races and geographic regions was the object of the evaluation. The regionalized perinatal care programs were intended to identify high-risk pregnancies and infants, for which proper management is offered. The end results of these programs are evaluated in the form of perinatal and postnatal mortality, maternal and newborn morbidity, and infant developments.

The method proposed by Gillings consists of the following steps:

- A trend line is fitted to the yearly plots of mortality so that the trend could be described by a smooth line. The statistical tool used is that of least squares.
- Each time period is represented by a separate linear trend called *segment*.
- Time trends for both the program and control areas are plotted. The schematic representation in Figure 5–1 has five segments for the program area and five for the control area. The program area had higher mortality than the control area, which could have been the basis for its selection to receive the program.
- Six parameters are characterized: (1) the intercept for segment 1, or the mean mortality in 1935 (β_0); (2) the slope of segment 1, or the linear trend between 1935 and 1945 (β_1); (3) the difference in slopes between segments 1 and 2 (β_2); (4, 5, and 6) the differences in slopes between subsequent segments (β_3, β_4, and β_5, respectively).
- The linear trends from one segment to another may be similar, meaning that $\beta_2 = \beta_3 = \beta_4 = \beta_5 = 0$. This forms the basis for the null hypothesis, which is tested by regression methods.
- The differences between the program and control regions are evaluated by tests of statistical significance. For example, the difference between the slopes of segment 3 is not statistically significant, which means that the program and control regions were similar before the program. Differences in the slopes begin to emerge for segments 4 and 5, which occur after the initiation of the program.
- In addition to performing the preceding analysis for the entire program and control regions, similar analyses may be performed within various age, sex,

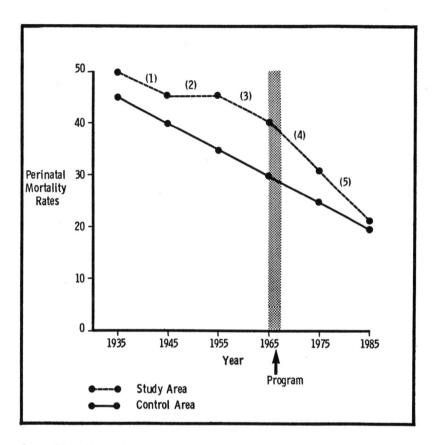

Source: Adapted from D. Gillings, D. Makuc, and E. Siegel, "Analysis of Interrupted Time Series Mortality Trends: An Example to Evaluate Regionalized Perinatal Care," *American Journal of Public Health* 71(1): 38–46.

Figure 5–1 Schematic Representation of Interrupted Time Series Analysis

race, etc., groups. The results of these analyses would strengthen the weight of the evidence.

These analyses have provided a historical review of the downward trend in perinatal mortality rates that would not have been otherwise recognized. Differences and similarities between the program and control areas have been documented. Although cause and effect may not be inferred with certainty, analysis of time trends offers a way of examining the possible impact of a program on a health state of a defined population without the considerable expenses of collecting primary data. This time series analysis employs ecologic procedures in which data are expressed in terms of the group's or entity's experience rather than the individual's. Regionalization is a concept that has been applied to a number of contiguous geographic (or county) units where certain barriers to health care have been removed. Infant and maternal mortality rates are overall indices reflecting the potential benefit of regionalization for populations in the geographic areas.

Another ecologic analysis was found useful in associating the length of response times to level of demand for emergency medical services (Mayer 1981). Geographical variations in mean response times within Seattle ranged from 1 minute in the city's downtown area to more than 11 minutes in several peripheral locations. Although the mean response time conforms to federal standards, ecologic correlations between response time and demand should provide interesting evidence for policy making. Demand was measured by the proxy of the number of emergency calls originating in a given area. Negative correlations mean that higher demand is associated with shorter response time. Geographic units incongruous with this general relationship would invite closer examination for developing an appropriate action.

TIME TRENDS AND MODELING

Modeling in this context refers to the collection and organization of information for a condition and its associated factors over time. This information in conjunction with outcome variables is analyzed in such a fashion that rates (mortality or morbidity) are obtained to represent expected values. That is, these rates are to be expected if "normal" forces prevail without any specific intervention. Expected rates may be adjusted by conventional statistical techniques for factors that are known to affect the "crude" rates. The potential influence of certain interventions on the improvements of a condition may be judged by comparing observed to expected rates. The percentage resulting from dividing the percentage of decrease in the *expected* rate of the condition from the beginning to the end of a period by the percentage of decrease in the corresponding *observed* rates gives an estimate of the contribution of the factor for which adjustment has been made. The balance of the percentage may be attributed to the influence of other factors including intervention measures.

Rh immune globulin (Rhogam) has been used in the United States since 1968 to prevent the condition known as *hemolytic disease of the newborn*. The immune globulin is given to Rh-negative mothers who run the risk of becoming sensitized by Rh-positive fetus. The immune globulin is given immediately after birth of the first child to prevent the disease in subsequent children. There have been no controlled trials to evaluate the impact of this preventive measure on the occurrence of hemolytic disease of the newborn. The incidence of this condition has decreased 65% in the United States over a 10-year period since 1970. How much of this decline is due to the introduction of Rhogam, and how much is due to other factors? This question may be answered, at least in part, by a combination of time trends and modeling analysis.

Hemolytic disease of the newborn is characterized by profound anemia, enlarged spleen and liver, and jaundice. It usually results in stillbirth or death soon after delivery. It occurs in Rh-negative pregnant women with Rh-positive fetuses. The Rh-positive fetus stimulates the production of Rh antibodies in the mother. In a subsequent pregnancy with an Rh-positive fetus, the fetus's red blood cells may be destroyed by maternal antibodies, resulting in hemolytic disease of the newborn. It follows, therefore, that children of a first pregnancy are not affected. Before Rhogam prophylaxis, risk, while minimal in a first pregnancy, increased gradually with each pregnancy of an Rh-positive fetus. Rhogam, which is given to mothers within three days of delivery, offers passive immunization. The Rhogam destroys the Rh factor. The end result is that the mother will not produce antibodies against the factor, therefore resulting in safe subsequent pregnancies.

Hemolytic disease of the newborn is positively associated with birth order in that the higher the birth order, the greater the incidence of the disease. Incidence rates of hemolytic disease of the newborn by birth order in Connecticut ranged from 6 per 10,000 births for birth order of 1 in 1972 to a rate of 205 for birth order of 5 or higher (Adams et al. 1981). The corresponding incidence rates in 1977 were 8 and 72. Although the relationship to birth order was maintained in the later period, there has been a considerable decrease in the rate from birth order 1 to birth order 5 or higher (from 205 to 72) between the two periods. The relationship to birth order bears an added significance since the distribution of live births by birth order in the United States has shown dramatic changes for the fourth and higher births. The percentage of fourth and higher births was 18% in 1970 and 10% in 1978 (Adams 1981 et al.)

The effect of birth order changes on the decline of the incidence of the hemolytic disease of the newborn may be computed as follows. An expected incidence rate of the disease for the United States in 1970 and 1978 is computed using conventional adjustment methods. These expected rates represent the rates that would have occurred had the birth order distribution between 1970 and 1978 not changed. The crude or observed rates for the same periods represent the actual rates, which include the effect of birth order distributions. Estimates of expected incidence rates for 1970 and 1978 were 50 and 39 respectively, representing a difference of 11 per 10,000, or a 22% decline (11 ÷ 50). The corresponding crude incidence rates of the disease in the United States in 1970 were 41 per 10,000 and in 1978, 14 per 10,000—or a difference of 27 per 10,000, representing a decrease of 66% (27 ÷ 41). Therefore, it can be estimated that about 33% (.22 ÷ .66) of the decrease in the incidence rates of hemolytic disease of the newborn from 1970 to

1978 may be due to changes in the birth order distribution (Adams et al. 1981). Therefore, it may be assumed that the remainder of the decrease—that is, 67% (100 − 33)—may be attributed largely to the impact of Rhogam.

In a more elaborate analysis on data from England and Wales for an earlier period (1961–73), the relative contributions of important factors to the decline in stillbirths and deaths from hemolytic disease of the newborn were investigated (Knox 1976). The stillbirths and deaths from hemolytic disease in the newborn per 1,000 births declined from a rate of 1.3 in 1961 to 0.5 in 1973, representing an average annual decline of 7.5%. The contribution of the shift in parity distribution over time must be taken into consideration in explaining the decrease. After adjustments for parity distributions by methods similar to those described, it was concluded that parity accounted for about 38% of the decline in stillbirths and deaths due to hemolytic disease of the newborn over the period under study.

What are the causes of the remaining 62% of the decline? A set of factors, possibly playing a minor role, was considered. The increase of women of non-European origin in whom the proportion of Rh negative is fewer than the 15% commonly found in European women, the increase in family planning and sterilization procedures, the changes in the incidence of toxemias of pregnancy, and the changes in the application of Caesarean section may have caused some of the decline of the stillbirths and deaths from hemolytic disease of the newborn. The contribution of all these factors was about 7%. Therefore about 45% of the decline has been explained.

Second, an important factor of nonspecific improvement in the general quality of medical care was considered. Examination of the stillbirth rate from *all* causes between 1961 and 1973 revealed about 35% reduction (from a rate of 19 to a rate of 12 per 1,000 total births). When all causes are considered, this reduction showed only a small variation by causes of stillbirth other than hemolytic disease of the newborn, and parity explains a small portion of the reduction. In other words it may be safe to assume that the 35% reduction in stillbirth could be attributed to general improvements in the quality of medical care.

About 80% of the decline has thus been explained primarily by shifts in parity distributions and improved quality of general medical care. The remaining 20% of the decline may be attributed to the immune globulin usage. In England and Wales between 1961 and 1973, the immune globulin was used only by about 5% of the women who were Rh-negative with Rh-positive fetuses. In the 1970s and beyond, the contribution of the Rhogam would be greater than 20%, as in the United States.

CLINICAL COURSE AND MODELING

The clinical course of a disease depends on a number of factors such as the physical, emotional, and psychologic status of the patient before the occurrence of the condition; the degree of severity of the condition and associated comorbidity; availability, accessibility, and quality of medical care; and the type of facility where the patient is finally placed. All these factors contribute to survival or death and to good or poor functional status. Such characteristics may be subjected to multivariate analysis to identify the responsible variables and quantify their effect on an end result such as survival with good functioning. This set of relationships provides a model of expected probabilities for specified events.

The case of the hip fracture provides an illustrative example (Zimmer 1975). The probability of a good functional status outcome according to levels of several factors was computed from records on 500 fractured hip cases. In addition, multivariate analysis identified three characteristics highly related to good outcome. These characteristics accounted for about one-third of the variance in the end result and included prefracture functional state, patient age, and complications. The relative importance to the outcome was given weights of 1, 2, and 3, respectively (Table 5–1). When the sum of the products of multiplying the probability of good functional outcome for a certain characteristic by the corresponding weight is divided by the sum of weights, an expected probability of good functional outcome for these characteristics is obtained. From the table, the expected probability of good functional outcomes for a person of good prefracture functional status who is 60 years of age and has no complication will be 0.80 (.89 × 1 + .76 × 2 + .80 × 3 ÷ 1 + 2 +3).

This model may be used to evaluate the impact of intervention programs. For example, if a new maneuver were applied to a group of patients who are 55 to 64 years of age, in good condition, and without complications, a good functional outcome should occur in better than 80% of the cases for the manuever to be declared successful. The gain above what is to be expected (80%) should, of course, be statistically significant and clinically meaningful.

In another example expected perinatal mortality rates were computed for 504 California hospitals (Williams 1979). The observed rate for each hospital was expressed in relation to the expected rate in an observed/expected index to reveal discrepancies in the rates. The effectiveness of perinatal medical care programs may be evaluated in reference to narrowing the gap between observed and expected rates. Successful programs would result in rates that exceed expectations.

In a final example the clinical course of coronary heart disease may be plotted. Risk factors to disease development, alternative methods of medical care, and cost estimates of each procedure in relation to an end result of survival and good quality of life may be quantified from available data (Sidel, Acton, Lown 1969). Decisions include screening of the population for risk factors; application of intervention measures; use of ambulance, mobile coronary care units, or community triage centers for patients; admission of patients to a coronary intensive care unit or regular hospital; and early or late hospital discharge. Numerical probabilities for

Table 5–1 The Probability of Good Functioning Outcome for Specified Characteristics

Characteristic	Probability	Weight
Prefracture state		1
good	0.89	
poor	0.11	
Age		2
<55	0.78	
55–64	0.76	
65–74	0.45	
75–84	0.35	
85+	0.24	
Complications		3
None	0.80	
Insignificant	0.53	
Single	0.42	
Multiple	0.18	

Source: Adapted from J.G. Zimmer and D. Puskin, "An Epidemiological Model of the Natural History of a Disease within a Multilevel Care System," *International Journal of Epidemiology* 4(2): 93–104.

these characteristics and measures, their consequences, and their costs may be obtained from available data. The result would be a set of relationships or a model of expected values. When a new procedure is introduced to a specific group of individuals at a specific stage of the clinical course, the observed outcome is compared with the expected outcome, therefore providing a means of evaluation of the new procedure.

Time trends, ecologic analyses, and modeling are useful techniques for describing and evaluating intervention programs. The evidence derived from these methods depends on the quality of the data used. Nevertheless, such methods are subject to potential selection bias. Selective factors that determine the allocation of treatment or programs to particular individuals or groups cannot be ignored in interpreting the results of this approach. Confounding factors are less serious since many of them could be taken into account in data analysis by stratification or adjustment techniques.

CONCLUSION

Time trends, ecologic correlations, and modeling are useful methods of evaluating health programs. They are attractive because they take advantage of published information, but the impact of factors other than the program of interest may limit the interpretation of the results.

Nevertheless, these methods have been used in assessing the impact of regionalized perinatal programs on reducing infant and maternal mortality, immune globulin on preventing hemolytic disease of the newborn, and alternate methods of medical care on survival from coronary heart disease.

BIBLIOGRAPHY

Adams MM, Marks JS, Gustafson J et al: Rh hemolytic disease of the newborn: Using incidence observations to evaluate the use of Rh immune globulin. *Am J Public Health* 1981; 71: 1031–1035.

Gillings D, Makuc D, Seigel E: Analysis of interrupted time series mortality trends: An example to evaluate regionalized perinatal care. *Am J Public Health* 1981; 71(1): 38–46.

Knox EG, Control of hemolytic disease of the newborn. *Brit J Prev Soc Med* 1976; 30: 163–169.

Mayer JD: A method for the geographical evaluation of emergency medical service performance. *Am J Public Health* 1981; 71(8): 841–844.

Sidel VW, Action, Lown: Models for the evaluation of prehospital coronary care. *Amer J Cardiol* 1969; 24: 674–688.

Williams, RL: Measuring the effectiveness of perinatal medical care. *Medical Care* 1979; 17(2): 95–111.

Zimmer JG, Puskin D: An epidemiological model of the natural history of a disease within a multilevel care system. *Intern J Epid* 1975; 4(2): 93–104.

Chapter 6

Case-Control, Before-After, and Cohort Studies

Case-control, before-after, and cohort studies are observational methods of investigations usually designed with a specific research question or hypothesis in mind. Since many potential biases can be taken into account in the design phase, these studies are in a better position than the time trends and modeling approaches in the hierarchy of research methods, as discussed in Chapter 4.

CASE-CONTROL STUDIES

The *case-control study* is that "method of epidemiological investigation in which the frequency of an attribute or exposure to an environmental factor in cases (individuals with a disease or another defined adverse health outcome) is compared to that in noncases or controls" (Ibrahim and Spitzer 1979, p. 139). That definition has been useful when the case-control study is used to investigate the possible causes of a disease—the traditional usage of epidemiologic investigations. For the purposes of health services research and policy, the *case-control study* may be defined as that method of epidemiological investigation in which the frequency of exposure to or utilization of health services in individuals who might have benefited from the service (cases) is compared with that in noncases or controls. As in other case-control studies, the difference in the two frequencies is tested for statistical significance and is used to calculate measures of relative and attributable risk (or benefit) in relation to nonexposure or nonuse to the health service activity in question.

The case-control approach has been a major tool in the evaluation of potential hazards of drugs such as the antihypertensive drug Reserpine and the hormone estrogen and their possible connections to breast cancer and uterine cancer, respectively. Such studies have received wide publicity and have had profound impact on health care practice. The relative ease with which case-control studies are undertaken increases its attractiveness for use as a basis for health policy. It is for these reasons that the potentials and limitations of this research strategy must become thoroughly understood by all concerned.

Pap testing has been in wide use for decades to discover cervical cancer in its early or preinvasive stage. The benefit of the test has not been conclusively shown since randomized, controlled trials could not have been undertaken; they are impractical and perhaps unethical. Several observational studies have shown that Pap testing may have been useful in preventing invasive cervical cancer. A case-control study was specifically designed to assess the effectiveness of Pap smear screening (Clarke and Anderson 1979). Newly diagnosed invasive cervical cancer cases in 212 women who were 20 to 69 years old formed the case group. These cases were of 323 eligible women who resided in the Toronto area and were admitted to Princess Margaret Hospital between 1 October 1973 and 30 September 1976. Non-respondents—111 cases, or 34%—were distributed between deaths, too ill to be interviewed, non-English speakers, or simple refusals. There is a potential of selection bias as a result of the high nonresponse rate.

The control group was matched on age within 10 years of the cases and in the ratio of five controls to one case. In order to reduce the potential confounding bias of socioeconomic status, the controls were chosen from the same neighborhood and type of dwelling as those of the cases.

Interviews were conducted at home for both cases and controls. Histories of Pap smear screening were obtained from study subjects in conjunction with physician visits as to whether the test was done routinely (as a preventive measure) or in response to symptoms. These histories were verified against physician records.

During the five years before the cancer diagnosis, 32% of the cases reported having one or more Pap smear tests compared to 56% of the controls. This difference "indicated a relative risk of invasive cancer of 2.7 in women who had not been screened by Pap smear, compared with those who had" (Clarke and Anderson 1979, p. 1). As discussed in Chapter 4, the relative risk is obtained by dividing the rate of the disease among the exposed by the rate of the disease among the nonexposed. It cannot be computed directly in case-control studies but may be approximated by the odds ratio which is calculated from the proportions of health service use in the cases and the controls.

The risk of developing invasive cervical cancer that is associated with not having Pap smear test is almost three times greater than the risk associated with having the test. The relative risk in case-control studies is computed as follows:

$$\frac{\text{Number of cases without test} \times \text{Number of controls with test}}{\text{Number of cases with test} \times \text{Number of controls without test}} = \frac{145 \times 591}{67 \times 469} = 2.7$$

In spite of the controls being matched on cases as to age and socioeconomic status, the control group were slightly younger, were better educated, and had a higher total family income. These factors are known to be associated with a Pap smear screening test as well as less likelihood of cervical cancer. Therefore, these factors may be a source of confounding bias. The association between socioeconomic status and the frequency of Pap smear screening was evident in this study in both the case and control group. Cases and controls were analyzed by age and sociodemographic specific groupings (stratification analysis) to control for potential confounding bias. This analysis revealed a relative risk of 2 or higher in those who failed to receive a Pap smear screening test.

Another confounding variable may be access to medical care, in that the low frequency of Pap smears in the cases may reflect fewer opportunities to see a physician. To consider this possible bias, data were reanalyzed for cases and controls who had seen a doctor at least once during the five years preceding the cancer diagnosis. The relative risk still held.

Finally, a confounding factor may be that of hysterectomies among controls. Control patients who have had hysterectomies would not be eligible for obtaining Pap smear screening. If these control patients were to be removed from the analysis (the denominator of the control group would be less), it would follow that a larger or smaller percentage of the control patients would have had Pap smear screenings, depending on whether patients had to be deleted from the numerator— those with both hysterectomies and Pap tests. The difference between controls and cases may therefore increase or decrease.

Another potential bias commonly found in case-control studies is that of selection. This bias is due to the "differential selection of subjects into the cases or control groups, resulting in a distorted measure of association or effect" (Ibrahim and Spitzer 1970, p. 141). Selection bias would be reduced if all or a random sample of all types of a disease in a defined area is included in the study. Representativeness would enhance the generalizability of the findings. In spite of the fact that cervical cancer cases in this study were derived from only one hospital, 80% of the cases in that community were first treated at that hospital. Therefore, representativeness might be reasonably assumed.

The representative issue is not widely advocated by scientists. Some believe that well-defined entities of cases may be the subject of investigation in a given study rather than a representative group of cases (Cole 1979). In this study the nonresponse rate was relatively high, 34%. Comparison of respondents with nonrespondents revealed similar percentages of patients who have had a Pap smear test before the first symptom, which is indicative that nonresponse selection bias may not be large.

Finally, information bias is the third type of bias commonly encountered in case-control studies. It occurs when information on cases, controls, or exposure variables is unknown or inaccurate, therefore resulting in misclassifications. These misclassifications could distort the measures of risk. A subtype of information bias is that of recall by the case in which past experiences are overestimated.

Another is an interviewer bias, in which the interviewer may report an exaggerated experience for a case, especially if the interviewer knows who is a case and who is a control subject. Analysis of recorded data would help identify the existence of information bias. In the cervical cancer study, recorded data provided similar relative risks as those obtained from information data.

Attributable risk is a measure of potential impact of programs on health states of populations. Attributable risk estimates have been computed from the findings of the cervical cancer study (Table 6–1). For example, 63% of cervical cancer risk may be attributed to no Pap smear tests in women who were not screened. In other words 63% of the invasive cervical cancers in unscreened women would have been prevented had they been screened. This attributable risk percentage measure should be useful for health planners and policy makers in deciding whether to introduce or fund a specific program.

BEFORE-AFTER STUDIES

Perhaps one of the easiest, but less satisfactory, methods of investigation of the impact of a program is to measure an end result before and after a specific program

Table 6–1 Measures of Potential Impact of Cervical Cancer Screening

Measure	Formula	Impact
Attributable risk	Relative risk − 1 $2.7 - 1 = 1.7$	An excess risk of 1.7 may be attributed to not having had Pap smear in women who were not screened, i.e., the amount of risk that is greater than expected (in women who have had the test).
Attributable risk percentage	$\dfrac{\text{Relative risk} - 1}{\text{Relative risk}} \times 100$ $\dfrac{2.7 - 1}{2.7} \times 100 = 63\%$	63% of cervical cancer risk may be attributed to not having had Pap smears in women who were not screened, i.e., 63% of cancers in these women would have been prevented if they had had the test.
Population attributable risk percentage	Proportion of Attributable women not × risk having test percentage $.4 \times 63\% = 25\%$	If the proportion of women not screened is .4, then 25% of the cervical cancer risk in all women may be attributed to not having had the test, i.e., 25% of all cervical cancers would have been prevented if all women had the test.

has been in operation. When the health states of a population change dramatically after a specific program, it is not too unreasonable to attribute the benefits to the particular program. For example, the dramatic decline in the number of cases of pertussis since 1945, poliomyelitis since 1955, measles since 1963, and rubella and mumps since about 1970 can be safely attributed to the immunization programs introduced for these diseases at the respective times. Such dramatic changes over a relatively short time in health states are the exception rather than the rule, and therefore most before-after studies do not generally provide evidence as conclusive as the one presented by these conditions.

The effectiveness of comprehensive care programs in Baltimore's Inner City was evaluated by the study of their effect on the incidence of rheumatic fever (Gordis 1973). Annual incidence of hospitalized first attacks of rheumatic fever in the 5- to 14-year-old black children residing in census tracts eligible for these programs was computed for the period 1968–70. Similar data were obtained for the period 1960–64, which preceded the comprehensive care programs. Two control groups were used: (1) children in adjacent but not eligible census tracts and (2) children living in nonadjacent and noneligible census tracts.

The analysis showed that hospitalizations for rheumatic fever have decreased 60% in the census tracts where the programs were introduced in comparison to other areas (Table 6–2). This study and its results may form the basis of some important questions, as discussed in Chapter 1. Similar questions may be raised in conjunction with this study as follows:

- Have the services (those of the comprehensive care program) been provided? Apparently they have, but documentation of this would have been desirable.
- Did the changes occur? The changes that would form the link between the program activities and the desired end result would have been increased use of medical care. Indirect evidence may be derived from the fact that about 95% of eligible children to the C and Y (Children and Youth) project were

Table 6–2 Annual Hospitalizations per 100,000 for First Attacks of Rheumatic Fever before and after the Program

	Before	*After*	*% of Change*
Program tracts	26.8	10.6	− 60.4
Adjacent tracts	18.1	15.3	− 15.5
Nonadjacent tracts	8.1	14.6	+ 80.0

Source: Adapted from L. Gordis, et al. "Effectiveness of Comprehensive-Care Programs Preventing Rheumatic Fever," *New England Journal of Medicine* 289 (22): 331–335.

registered (Gordis 1973). This is helpful although registration does not imply usage.

- Have the objectives of the programs been achieved, and were the results convincing to policy makers? Before-after studies are usually conducted after the fact and not as a planned effort for timely input into policy making.
- Can the observed changes be attributed to the program? There might, of course, have been considerable changes in the social and economic conditions of the population between the two periods. These changes could have been responsible for the improvement noted in the incidence of hospitalizations for rheumatic fever. The incidence of hospitalizations was further analyzed according to whether the rheumatic fever attacks were preceded by clinical respiratory infections. Clinical respiratory infections are the main trigger for initiating therapy and therefore would be indicative of the influence of preventive measure rather than social change. A decline of 52% occurred in the hospitalizations in which attacks of rheumatic fever were preceded by respiratory infections, with no change in the cases without prior respiratory infections. Since the essence of the preventive program is the prompt recognition and treatment of infection, the analysis according to the presence of prior infection is an excellent technique to answer the question of social versus medical care influence.

Before-after studies may be strengthened by refinements such as

- documentation of environmental and socioeconomic changes over time, which may have influenced the outcome;
- correction for expected improvements due to regression toward the mean;
- comparison with the experiences of one or more control groups;
- use of several measurements rather than simply one before and one after the program, allowing for the confirmation of a trend consistent with the expected achievements by the program;
- analysis by the amount of service to reveal a dose-response relationship;
- review of the experiences of similar programs conducted by different investigators and in different settings, using different methodologies—replication of findings strengthens the conclusions; and
- control for potential confounding and selective biases in the analysis by proper techniques.

In another before-after study, the distributions of medical services before and after a government-sponsored insurance program for physician services in Montreal were analyzed (Enterline et al. 1973). Physician visits, symptoms, waiting times, and patient satisfaction were used as end results. Household members of a random half of 6,000 dwelling units were interviewed in the period before the program, and members of the other half were interviewed in the period after the program. No control group was used. The results showed a marked shift in the number of physician visits from individuals in the higher to the lower socioeconomic groups. The proportion of certain symptoms for which a doctor was visited also increased in the lower economic groups. A lengthening of waiting times was noted in the higher economic groups. The majority of patients considered the care satisfactory.

This study answers two important questions with relation to the compulsory insurance program. Did the insurance program increase accessibility to medical care by lower economic groups, and has the increased accessibility been used properly by them? It would seem that the program has achieved its purpose in that it removed financial barriers of accessibility and resulted in increased physician visits by the lower economic groups, that is, democratization of accessibility of medical care. In addition, the percentage of important symptoms for which a physician was seen increased among the lower economic groups after the insurance program was instituted. This finding emphasized the fact that physician visits were initiated for important symptoms, implying proper use of the increased accessibility. This study is important with regard to policies for health care insurance and medical care administration generally. It is not "epidemiologic" in that it does not address the question of impact on the health status of the populations of either economic group as a result of the insurance program.

COHORT STUDIES

Cohort studies refer to the analysis of the events in a group of individuals who have a common experience such as a birth date (a birth cohort). If one segment of the cohort has been exposed to a program and the other has not or has been exposed to a different program, comparison of the results between the two cohort segments may thus be made. The strength of this analysis is in its prospective nature and, depending on the type of data and the question asked, confounding and information biases may be minimal. Selection bias remains a potential problem since a subsegment of the cohort is offered a program because of known or unknown selective factors. This potential selective bias should be evaluated carefully before conclusions are reached.

Prenatal care and pregnancy outcome in a prepaid medical plan were compared with those in the general population (Quick, Greenlick, and Roghmann 1981). The experiences of more than 19,000 births in Portland in 1972–74 were compared with those of more than 4,000 births among members of the Kaiser-Permanente Medical Care Group of Portland. Birth certificates of 1973–74 formed the basis of data, and death certificates for infants for the years 1973–75 were matched with birth records. Information on prenatal care, sociodemographic risks, and medical obstetric risks on the mother was obtained from the birth certificate.

The relationship between prenatal care and prematurity in the presence or absence of risk in the mother is once more documented (Table 6–3). A prenatal care index, based on the month in which prenatal care began and the frequency of prenatal care visits adjusted for gestational age, ranged from 1 (adequate) to 3 (inadequate). Mothers may be classified into having no risks at all or having sociodemographic or medical obstetrical risks. Prematurity increased in both the no-risk and risk mother category as the quality of prenatal care worsened from adequate to inadequate. In the absence of risk the prematurity rate increased from 1.9 in the adequate care category, to 3.3 in the intermediate care category, and to 4.3 in the inadequate care category. When risk was present, a similar gradient was observed. Within each level of prenatal care, prematurity increased when risk was present. That is, prematurity was related to both sociodemographic and medical obstetrical risks in mothers as well as the quality of prenatal care received.

Prepaid medical care plans have been considered by some not as good as regular care because it is assumed that prepaid plans compromise quality to reduce costs. The Kaiser-Permanente experience presented here and that of the Health Insurance Plan of Greater New York (Shapiro et al. 1960) have shown otherwise. Neonatal and infant deaths in the Kaiser-Permanente group compared favorably with the general population (Table 6–4). In the presence of medical-obstetrical risk or both

---

Table 6–3 Prenatal Care and Percentage of Prematurity by Sociodemographic and Medical-Obstetrical Risk in the Oregon Population

Sociodemographic and Medical-Obstetrical Risk	Prenatal Care Index[a]		
	1	2	3
No risk	1.9	3.3	4.3
Risk present	9.8	15.8	21.4

[a]A measure of prenatal care calculated from the month in which prenatal care began and the frequency of visits, adjusted for gestational age (1 = adequate, 2 = intermediate, 3 = inadequate).

Source: Adapted from J.D. Quick, M.R. Greenlick, and K.J. Roghmann, "Prenatal Care and Pregnancy Outcome in an HMO and General Population: A Multivariate Cohort Analysis," *American Journal of Public Health* 71(4): 381–390.

sociodemographic and medical-obstetrical risks, the neonatal and infant death rates were less in the HMO group than in the general population.

These favorable results for the HMO could not have been attributed to prenatal care since the proportion of HMO women who visited physicians in the first trimester of pregnancy was less than that of women in the general population. The potential effect of confounding of the mothers' risk status has been considered and largely discounted by the stratification analysis. Since prematurity was associated with prenatal care (Table 6–3), the favorable results exhibited by the HMO population could not have been confounded by prematurity. It would seem reasonable to infer, therefore, that the pregnancy outcome in prepaid medical care plans of the Kaiser-Permanente and the Health Insurance Plan of Greater New York is as good as that in other systems of medical care. Others may want to say it is even better. In either case the information is crucial for policy development with reference to this form of medical care delivery system.

CONCLUSION

Case-control, before-after, and cohort are observational studies usually designed to answer a specific research question or test a hypothesis. The case-control approach has been used to assess the effectiveness of preinvasive cervical

---

Table 6–4 Neonatal and Infant Deaths per 1,000 Live Births by Risk Group, General and HMO Population

Risk Category	Neonatal Deaths		Infant Deaths	
	General Population	HMO	General Population	HMO
No risk	2.1	3.8	5.4	5.1
Sociodemographic risk	2.5	14.2	10.8	28.5
Medical-obstetrical risk	21.1	16.1	25.8	19.5
Sociodemographic and medical-obstetrical risk	22.8	20.6	30.6	26.5
All groups	9.2	9.4	13.9	12.5

Source: Adapted from J.D. Quick, M.R. Greenlick, and K.J. Roghmann, "Prenatal Care and Pregnancy Outcome in an HMO and General Population: A Multivariate Cohort Analysis," *American Journal of Public Health* 71(4): 381–390.

cancer screening programs. The impact of preventive programs on the incidence of rheumatic fever in an inner city population was evaluated by a before-after analysis. The cohort design proved useful in examining prenatal care and pregnancy outcomes in a prepaid medical care plan.

In all these approaches, selection, confounding, and information biases must be carefully considered. Societal changes or demographic characteristics that might impact on the outcome should be described and analyzed. Stratification analysis in the search for consistency and revelation of special effects is particularly useful.

BIBLIOGRAPHY

Clarke EA, Anderson TW: Does screening by "Pap" smears help prevent cervical cancer? A case-control study. *Lancet* July 7, 1979, pp 1–4.

Cole P: The evolving case-control study. *J Chron Dis* 1979; 32: 15–27.

Enterline PE, Salter V, McDonald AD et al: The distribution of medical services before and after "free" medical care—The Quebec experience. *N Engl J Med* 1973; 289(22): 1174–1178.

Gordis L: Effectiveness of comprehensive-care programs in preventing rheumatic fever. *N Engl J Med* 1973; 289(22): 331–335.

Ibrahim MA, Spitzer WO: The case-control study: The problem and the prospect. *J Chron Dis* 1979; 32: 139–144.

Quick JD, Greenlick MR, Roghmann KJ: Prenatal care and pregnancy outcome in an HMO and general population: A multivariate cohort analysis. *Am J Public Health* 1981; 71(4): 381–390.

Shapiro S, Jacobziner H, Densen PM et al: Further observations on prematurity and perinatal mortality in a general population and in a population of a prepaid medical care plan. *Am J Public Health* 1960; 50: 1304–1317.

Chapter 7

Randomized Controlled Trials

*Rational decisions at all levels in health care—from federal govern-
ment policy making to the treatment of a single patient by a physician—
require sound information. Randomized clinical trials (RCTs), a family
of clinical experimental designs, provide the highest quality of evidence
for the efficacy and safety of medical technologies.*

U.S. Congress, Office of Technology Assessment

The growing importance of randomized trials as the scientific method for
providing firm conclusions about the beneficial or harmful effects of health
programs stems from several reasons. Skepticisms are often voiced about accepting clinical or public health procedures on the basis of anecdotal information or
observational methods of study. These skepticisms have been reinforced by the
increased role and interest of the federal government in determining the effectiveness of several procedures in order to set policy standards for payments.

As organizations mandated to develop standards of quality of care emerged,
such as the professional standard review organizations, so did the need for solid
evidence with regard to efficacy and effectiveness of methods of care. Three
additional developments have been happening. First, methods of research design,
data analysis, and computing technology have improved and become widely
available. Second, epidemiology as an investigative science in the search for
causes of disease and as an applied science for the planning and evaluation of
health services has become more popular and better understood by the public as
well as scientists other than epidemiologists. Finally, British scientists have had
some influence on American scientists by advocating randomized trials as a sound
method for drawing conclusions that are adequate for a basis of policy making.

Randomized trials may be clinically or community based. Randomized clinical trials are often used to test the superiority of a specific medical care activity, such as the use of drugs or performance of operations, over standard methods of treatment. Randomized clinical trials are performed in clinical settings and are designed to answer the question of efficacy, that is, the impact of the procedure on those who receive it. Examples include the evaluation of adult onset diabetes control by dietary means and one of four therapeutic regimens, or high blood pressure by stepped care programs of antihypertensive medications.

Randomized community trials are conducted in community settings and are designed to test the effectiveness and efficiency of a health care intervention program. Community trials address issues of relevance to the operation of the health care system such as organizations and costs. Questions of adherence, dropping out, psychosocial factors, and quality of life as they pertain to the intervention procedure itself and its consequences are also of concern. Community trials often deal with measures of changing a population's behaviors and are exemplified by testing the effectiveness of hypertension control by screening, detection, and follow-up programs in defined populations.

Randomized trials have been instrumental in setting policies for health care. Questions that could be answered by the randomized method would have far-reaching implications for the health care system. Examples include hospital-based versus ambulatory care, home-based care versus self-care, and surgical procedures versus medical treatment. If the medical treatment (by injections) is as good as surgical treatment of varicose veins, patients and possibly physicians may choose the medical option. Questions of the length of stay and ambulation of patients are of great interest to health care policy makers. Early discharge or ambulation of patients with heart attacks would impact on both patients' health state and cost of care. Firm evidence as to the impact of changing behavior toward dietary intake, smoking, exercise, and stress would provide the needed basis for introducing community level programs.

Three large-scale intervention trials conducted by the National Heart, Lung, and Blood Institute deserve special mention. The Lipid Research Clinics (LRC) trial involved 3,810 men from 12 centers where study subjects were recruited from the general population or through referrals from physicians and blood banks (Lipid Research Clinics Program 1984). It was designed to test the hypothesis that diet alone or diet and cholesterol-lowering drugs will result in reduction in coronary heart disease risk. The Multiple Risk Factor Intervention Trial (MRFIT) was conducted on 13,000 men in 20 centers (Multiple Risk Factor Intervention Trial Research Group 1982). Subjects were recruited through screening procedures conducted in industries and communities. The study was designed to test the impact of dietary modification, antihypertensive medication, and smoking cessation on reducing the risk from coronary heart disease.

The third national trial is that of the Hypertension Detection and Follow-Up Program (HDFP), which involved 10,940 men and women in 14 centers where study subjects were recruited as a result of community screening activities (Hypertension Detection and Follow-up Program Cooperative Group 1979). The study tested the impact of stepped antihypertensive care regimen in contrast to the usual form of care. These large-scale trials, with the exception of the MRFIT, showed that the treatment of hypertension and the lowering of blood cholesterol are associated with significant reductions in coronary heart disease risk.

SOME BASIC PRINCIPLES OF RCTs

The most important aspect of RCTs is the random allocation of subject to the treatment or control group. "The essence of such a trial is comparison . . . we need not only the group of patients to be submitted to a special treatment . . . but another group differently treated. . . . The first step . . . is the *random* allocation of patients to one or other of these groups" (Hill 1952, p. 115). The randomization takes the assignment of subjects into either group out of the hands of the investigators as well as the participants, thus removing potential selective factors from the decision of giving a particular form of treatment. In addition, randomization should provide two comparable groups, especially when the sample size is large. Therefore, observed differences between the two groups may be attributed to the actual effect of treatment or to chance resulting from sampling fluctuations. Chance may be ruled out as the cause of the difference with a stated probability (generally 5%) by the application of an appropriate statistical test of significance.

In order to guarantee two comparable groups on specific characteristics, the study population must be stratified on such characteristics in advance of the randomization. Random allocation of the two groups must then be made within each stratum. Stratification is desirable on prognostic factors that are known key variables predictive of the end results. A postrandomization test should be performed to ensure that the two groups are comparable. If the two groups are comparable, randomization has succeeded in producing two similar groups. If they are not comparable on certain key characteristics, or if there are reasons to believe that the outcome variable should be analyzed according to subgroups at various risk within each study group, appropriate stratification on one or more prognostic factors will be in order. These prognostic factors may be the degree of risk, level of functional capacity, or probability of survival. The end result variable is analyzed between comparable prognostic strata of the treatment and control groups.

Prognostic stratification offers two advantages. It increases statistical efficiency in that differences will be more likely to be revealed. The findings will not be "diluted" if there is a disproportionate contribution to the outcome variable of a particular stratum. Second, prognostic stratifications in health care research help to identify those subsets of individuals who would benefit most (or least) from a particular intervention. The results of a randomized controlled trial thus become more applicable to the problems of the real world of health care.

The value of randomization may be gleaned from comparison of studies in which randomized control groups versus historical control groups were used. In one example, in almost 80% of the studies in which historical control groups were used, the new therapy was found to be better than the standard treatment. This is in contrast to only 20% of the experiments in which the control groups were randomized (Sacks, Chalmers, and Smith 1982). Another group of 145 studies was divided into 57 studies in which the randomization process was blinded, 45 in which it might have been unblinded, and 43 in which the controls were selected by nonrandom process (Chalmers et al. 1983). Differences in case fatality rates between treatment and control groups were found in only 9% of the blinded randomized studies in contrast to 25% of the unblinded randomized studies and 58% of the nonrandomized studies. These observations emphasize the pitfall of using nonrandomized control groups and unblinding the patient's status in that positive results may be due to potential biases introduced by these factors.

Another question in RCTs is the application of a fixed schedule of treatment or a varied regimen that depends on the patient's response and physician's judgment. Each approach answers a different question, which could determine the selection of one or the other approach. A varied drug regimen or home visitation schedule chosen according to the health care professional's judgment and patient's response would be more realistic but difficult to replicate. A fixed regimen would be easier to replicate but might not be completely applicable in the real world.

The nature of the outcome measure—mortality, morbidity, or disability— should be decided before beginning the trial. Unless the outcome is agreed a priori, objectivity of the investigator and confidence in the results may suffer. Masking or blinding of the investigators as to the correct placement of the study subject while assessing the outcome is important to prevent bias in collecting the information. This is obviously not crucial if the outcome is measured by entirely objective means.

Of ethical concern is the issue of exposing patients to a potentially hazardous procedure or denying them a potentially beneficial one. There would have been no need to perform the trial initially if the hazards or benefits were known. The trial is needed to find such consequences. Hazards are minimized by the critical appraisal of available information (on animals or people) and careful monitoring of patients during trial. Since one cannot deny a procedure that's perceived to be beneficial, the investigator with limited resources may stagger the trial in time or location, that is, offering the intervention to half of the subjects on a randomized basis, and after the results are documented and the procedure proves beneficial, the procedure may be offered to the other half.

Finally, it is known that large sample size and long periods of follow-up improve the accuracy of the results of RCTs and thereby increase the confidence and the chances of finding a difference, if in fact it does exist. Although this is desirable, longer follow-up periods and larger sample size cost money. A balance between cost and accuracy determines the proper course of action.

A NEW DESIGN FOR RANDOMIZED CONTROLLED TRIALS

It has been proposed, but not yet widely accepted, that controlled trials may be designed differently than at present (Zelen 1979). In the new design, study subjects are randomized to two groups A and B, where group A receives the standard treatment, and patients in group B are asked for their informed consent about accepting a new treatment. They would receive the standard treatment if they refuse, but they would receive the experimental treatment if they agree. Whereas informed consent occurs at step 2 in the conventional design, randomization occurs at step 2 in the Zelen design (Table 7–1). In the conventional design the results apply to groups A and B whose patients have already consented to participate in the trial. In the Zelen design, group A receiving the standard

---

Table 7–1 Differences between the Conventional and Zelen Designs of Randomized Controlled Trials

Conventional Design			Step	Zelen Design			
Study subjects			1	Study subjects			
Informed Consent			2	Randomization			
Yes	I	No			Group A I	Group B	
Randomization	I	—	3	No informed consent asked	I	Informed consent	
Group A I	Group B	—			I No	I Yes	
Standard I treatment	Experimental treatment	—	4	Standard treatment	I	Standard treatment	I Experimental treatment
Testing of results			5	Testing of results			

Source: Adapted from Figures 1 and 2, M. Zelen, "A New Design for Randomized Controlled Trials," *New England Journal of Medicine* 300 (22): 1242–1245.

treatment will be compared with group B regardless of whether patients in that group are receiving the standard or the experimental treatment.

One drawback of the Zelen design is the potential loss of statistical efficiency due to dilution of differences as a result of no improvement in group B patients who are receiving the standard treatment. Loss of statistical efficiency can be viewed from two different perspectives. First, the differences revealed between the two groups using the Zelen design will be revealed in spite of the possible dilution effect by those receiving standard treatment in group B. That is, inferences with regard to the superiority of the experimental treatment would be conservative. Second, the loss of statistical efficiency could be remedied by increasing the sample size appropriately.

Ethical issues raised by the Zelen design are those of not informing the patients assigned to the standard treatment that they are participating in a randomized trial and of using data generated by this group without informed consent (Zelen 1979). It could be argued that patients expect standard treatment anyway, and therefore there is no reason to obtain their informed consent. Since the data on the group receiving standard treatment will be analyzed and published in the aggregate without identification of individuals, it therefore does not differ from using aggregate data on patients or individuals in usual epidemiologic investigations.

SOME ISSUES IN HEALTH SERVICE RESEARCH

When patients are randomized into treatment and control groups to receive the treatment as a group, rather than as individuals as in the case of health education or prenatal care classes, certain practical problems may arise. What, for example, is the optimal size of a group suitable for health education classes? Experiences in group psychotherapy would indicate that a group composed of 8 to 12 individuals would be ideal for free discussions and exchange of experiences (Ibrahim et al. 1974; Ibrahim 1976). If there are several treatment groups, would different therapists or educators be used with the concomitant interobserver variability, or would the same therapist or educator be allowed to lead several groups? The latter approach would raise an issue of practicability since the same person may not be readily available to lead more than one group. Should men and women or persons of different backgrounds be included in one group, or should the group be homogeneous? Experiences with this kind of research indicate that a hetero-geneous group would be more interesting and conducive to a free exchange of ideas than a homogeneous group would be.

In a group psychotherapy study for coronary heart disease patients (Ibrahim et al. 1974; Ibrahim 1976) questions arose as to the impact of deaths of group members on the rest of the patients. Problems may arise as the result of possible conflicting advice to patients of different physicians. Finally, what happens with the cost of the therapy? It appeared that members of the group develop cohesion and self-support sufficient to cope with the problem of the death of a member. Since every patient, even with the same symptoms, is different from any other patient, the problems of receiving different advice from physicians were interpreted in that light. Finally, a group of 10 patients receiving treatment once a week costs only a few hundred dollars per year per patient, which would be affordable.

Could group sessions be conducted without a leader or therapist? This would obviously reduce the costs, but good dynamics and free interactions may not be fostered without a leader. Would a former patient serve as a group leader rather than a psychotherapist? This is possible but would need to be tested. A final question on these types of studies is the possible inclusion of spouses since, at least in coronary heart disease, changes in life style of one member of the spouse pair would usually involve the other member. Spouses have been included in the group in some studies, but the research experience is insufficient to arrive at definitive conclusions on this issue.

DESCRIPTION OF RANDOMIZED CLINICAL TRIALS

These trials are generally done on a defined clinic population that is first subjected to a series of tests and procedures to exclude ineligible patients, such as those with certain complications (Figure 7–1). A prerandomization period of about three months is spent assessing compliance with medication, side effects, and attendance records. Patients with such problems are identified and excluded. The remaining study subjects form the eligible pool of patients who are allocated to treatment or control groups by means of a randomization process using tables of random numbers or computer-generated random numbers. The control group receives the standard treatment or placebo, and the other treatment group receives the promising drug or new technology. The end result is measured in individuals in the two groups, and differences are tested by appropriate statistical tests. Sample size is determined in advance of the trial so that a statistically significant difference with a known probability can be obtained.

An important question in randomized trials is that of ethical considerations in depriving a group from receiving the "promising" treatment. There is an ethical problem of denying a treatment that is perceived effective to patients forming the control group. On the other hand, if the treatment is promising, yet unproven, then the trial is needed to ensure that the new treatment is superior to the standard treatment. Complex ethical issues hinder the initiation of randomized trials.

The statistical power of a clinical trial is the probability of detecting a result of a specified magnitude at a specified level of significance. This statistical power is directly related to sample size in that as the sample size increases, so does the probability of detecting a designated result. A balance, of course, must be made

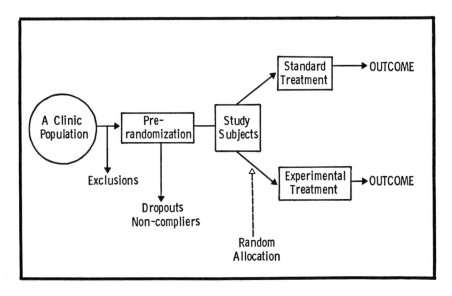

Figure 7–1 Randomized Clinical Trials

between the cost of a large sample size and the statistical power of finding a difference.

The approval of drugs and medical devices by the Food and Drug Administration relies heavily on the findings from randomized clinical trials. But once the drug or device is introduced, further trials are performed on a voluntary basis by scientists at large.

DESCRIPTION OF RANDOMIZED COMMUNITY TRIALS

After the efficacy of a new treatment, procedure, device, or health program has been shown in a tightly controlled clinical setting where the noncomplying, dropouts, and patients with side effects are excluded, the intervention may be tested at the community level. A *study population* is identified as a subset of a defined larger population. This study population is randomized to those receiving usual care and those receiving experimental care. The two groups receiving care are observed for end results as well as acceptance of the program, compliance with prescribed regimen, and emergence of side effects.

After a Community Trial

The role of epidemiology in health service research starts with epidemiologic studies of causation to identify risk factors, which together with epidemiologic methods of program evaluation form the basis of observational methods described in Chapters 5 and 6. After observational methods have given preliminary evidence of the potential benefits of an intervention, clinical trials may be in order, followed by community trials. After a specific intervention has been proven clinically and at the community level to be efficacious and effective, the intervention may be introduced in the form of a health program whereby the impact on the health state of the population is monitored and evaluated.

The cycle represents a logical sequence of events (Figure 7–2). In the real world, observational methods may or may not precede clinical or community trials, and often clinical and community trials are not done, making it necessary to initiate service programs on the basis of observational methods of evaluation. In other instances, health programs are introduced into the community without even observational evidence. Monitoring and surveillance of their potential impact on the health of populations are all that is left as a means of evaluation.

CASE EXAMPLES

An example of a randomized *clinical* trial may be seen in testing the effects of antihypertensive treatment on morbidity and mortality from hypertension (Veterans Administration Cooperative Study Group on Antihypertensive Agents 1970).

Patients included in this trial were male veterans who were hospitalized for hypertension (diastolic blood pressure 90–129 mm Hg). A prerandomization period of three months was the first step in the trial during which patients received placebos. During this period of observation, patients with severe hypertension complications, those who were unwilling or unable to honor the clinic schedule, and those who did not comply with the medication regimen were excluded. Since in a controlled *clinical* trial the main objective is to determine the efficacy of an intervention—in this case a medication—a prerandomization period of observation is an excellent way of excluding patients who would not contribute to the main aim of the trial. Compliance to medication was tested by the presence of a bright yellow fluorescence in the urine due to riboflavin that was incorporated in the placebo. Examination of urine specimens and counting pills afforded an opportunity to test the patient's reliability.

Patients with average diastolic blood pressure of 90 to 129 mm Hg were randomized to either an active drug or a placebo group. The placebos were

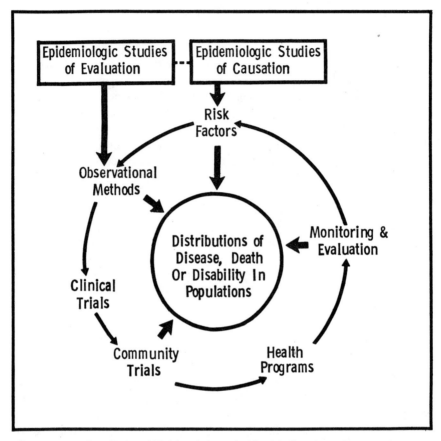

Figure 7–2 The Role of Epidemiology in Health Services Research

identical in taste and appearance to the active drugs. After three years of observation, patients in the control group with high levels of diastolic blood pressure (i.e., 115 to 129 mm Hg) experienced significantly higher morbid events. This required terminating the experiment for this group of patients and excluding them from further tests.

Clinic visits were scheduled at bimonthly intervals for the observation period. Elaborate annual examinations, which included x-rays of the chest and electrocardiograms, were performed on all participants.

Patients with diastolic blood pressures of 90 to 114 numbered 380 and formed the basis of the results in that study. In spite of randomization, the two groups were compared on prognostic factors in a postrandomization test for assessing whether randomization had truly worked. The two groups were found to be relatively comparable.

The first question was, Does blood pressure level change with medication? Systolic and diastolic blood pressures were reduced in the treated patients and remained at reduced levels throughout observation. Diastolic blood pressure, for example, fell about 17 mm Hg in the treated group compared with a rise of about 1 mm Hg in the control patients. The second question relates to the frequency of morbid events such as cerebral vascular accident, coronary heart disease, and congestive heart failure in the treated versus the nontreated group. The protection of treatment, analyzed by life table techniques, was shown to increase with time and continue throughout the five-year period of follow-up. The cumulative incidence of all morbid events in the control group rose to 55% compared with only 18% in the treated group.

A randomized *community* trial using a service rather than a drug was tested on patients discharged from a geriatric rehabilitation hospital (Nielson et al. 1972). Patients were randomly allocated to a group receiving home health aide services or to a group not receiving such services. Three end results were measured during a one-year period of follow-up: survival, contentment, and institutionalization.

Six individuals among the 50 participants in the service program died, compared with 4 in the 50 in the group with no service program—a statistically insignificant difference. Contentment, a measure of the quality of life, was documented by patient responses to four questions about happiness and life satisfaction and also by an observer rating. Favorable changes were noted in the service group and not in the control group. Patients who received the home aide service spent fewer days in institutions than patients who did not receive these services. Furthermore, fewer patients were admitted to institutions in the service group than in the control group. Additional analyses of subgroups within the two study groups revealed that certain patients, such as those with arthritis and those who might have a potential care-giver in the home, would benefit most from the intervention. The findings of this study provide preliminary information that might have implications for caring for elderly subjects.

A final example relates to the evaluation of services in a prepaid group practice by a controlled trial in which 1,580 persons were randomly assigned to a fee-for-service or to the Group Health Cooperative of Puget Sound (Manning et al. 1984). The hospitalization rate was 40% less and the expenditure rate for all services was 25% less at the cooperative than at the fee-for-service system. The inference was made that "the style of medicine at prepaid group practices is markedly less 'hospital-intensive' and, consequently, less expensive" (Manning et al. 1984). After several before-after and comparative studies showed that prepaid plans do not necessarily serve selected populations and that their impact on health states is similar to other systems, this randomized controlled trial offered firm evidence for substantial reductions in costs. A policy for a cost-effective system of care may be in the making.

CONCLUSION

Randomized controlled trials provide the firmest evidence for assessing the effects of a health program or a medical procedure. Randomized trials may be clinically or community based. While the former are performed in clinical settings and are designed to test efficacy, the latter are conducted in communities and are designed to answer questions of effectiveness and efficiency. Random allocation, stratification (pre- or postrandomization), a priori agreement on the outcome measure, and ethical issues are important considerations in the design and conduct of randomized trials.

The Veterans Administration randomized clinical trial offered firm evidence for the efficacy of antihypertensive medication. Later large-scale community trials answered questions of compliance, acceptance, and other issues of implementation of preventive programs in communities.

BIBLIOGRAPHY

Chalmers TC, Celano P, Sacks HS et al: Bias in treatment assignment in controlled clinical trials. *N Engl J Med* 1983; 309: 1358–1361.

Hill AB: The clinical trial. *N Engl J Med* 1952; 247(4): 113–119.

Hypertension Detection and Follow-up Program Cooperative Group: Five year findings of the hypertension detection and follow-up program: II. Mortality by race, sex and age. *JAMA* 1979; 242: 2572–2577.

Ibrahim MA: The impact of intervention upon psychosocial functions of postmyocardial infarction patients. *J S Carol Med Assoc* 1976; 72 (suppl): 23–26.

Ibrahim MA, Feldman JG, Sultz HA et al: Management after myocardial infarction: A controlled trial of the effect of group psychotherapy. *Int J Psychiat Med* 1974; 5(3): 253–268.

Lipid Research Clinics Program: The Lipid Research Clinics Coronary Primary Prevention Trial Results. *JAMA* 1984; 251: 351–374.

Manning WG, Leibowitz A, Goldberg GA et al: A controlled trial of the effect of a prepaid group practice on use of services. *N Engl J Med* 1984; 310: 1505–1510.

Multiple Risk Factor Intervention Trial Research Group: Multiple Risk Factor Intervention Trial: Risk factor changes and mortality results. *JAMA* 1982; 248: 1465–1477.

Nielson M, Blenkner M, Bloom M et al: Older persons after hospitalization: A controlled study of home aide service. *Am J Pub Health* 1972; 62(8): 1094–1101.

Sacks H, Chalmers TC, Smith H: Randomized versus historical controls for clinical trials. *Amer J Med* 1982; 72: 233–240.

US Congress, Office of Technology Assessment: The impact of randomized clinical trials on health policy and medical practice, background paper, publication No. OTA-BP-H-22, Government Printing Office, August 1983.

Veterans Administration Cooperative Study Group on Antihypertensive Agents: Effects of treatment on morbidity in hypertension: II. Results in patients with diastolic blood pressure averaging 90 through 114 mm Hg. *JAMA* 1970; 213 (7): 1143–1152.

Zelen M: A new design for randomized controlled trials. *N Engl J Med* 1979; 300(22): 1242–1254.

Part III

Preventive Services

Chapter 8

Health Promotion and Disease Prevention

An ounce of prevention is worth a pound of cure.

CHANGES IN LEADING CAUSES OF DEATH

The leading causes of death in the United States have changed dramatically from 1900 to 1980 (Table 8–1). The five leading causes of death in 1900 were ranked as follows: influenza and pneumonia, tuberculosis, diarrhea and related diseases, heart disease, and stroke. The first three causes of death were infectious in nature, while the chronic conditions of heart disease and stroke came fourth and fifth. The ranking of causes of death in 1980 is entirely different from 1900. Influenza and pneumonia rank as the fifth cause of death, while heart disease leads

Table 8–1 Leading Causes of Death in 1900 and 1980

1900	Rank	1980
Influenza and pneumonia	1	Heart disease
Tuberculosis	2	Malignant neoplasms
Diarrhea and related diseases	3	Stroke
Heart disease	4	Accidents, poisoning, & violence
Stroke	5	Influenza & pneumonia

Source: Adapted from Figure 5, National Center for Health Statistics, *Health, United States, 1980,* U.S. Department of Health and Human Services publication no. (PHS) 81–1232 (Washington, D.C.: U.S. Government Printing Office, December 1980).

the list. Malignant neoplasms, stroke, and accidents rank second, third, and fourth, respectively.

The control of infectious diseases has been achieved largely as a result of the application of health protection measures. These include changes in environmental conditions, water supply, and food products. These measures were taken at the point of origin, such as chlorination of water, pasteurization of milk, fortification of foodstuffs, and safe disposal of human waste. These interventions did not require individual action to effect the change. In fact, individuals were either passive or unaware while the interventions took place.

The other important factor responsible for the decline of infectious diseases over the years is immunization against childhood diseases. Immunization, a form of preventive health service requiring cooperation of individuals, has been the most effective preventive measure to date. The cooperation required is minimal and achieved by a limited number of visits to a health care professional to receive immunizations. In some instances, immunizations are required by law before entering the school system, in which case the individual generally has no choice but to cooperate and obey the law.

Unlike infectious diseases that were caused by known germs and were amenable to health protection or preventive health services, the causes of chronic diseases are generally unknown. Years of research have identified several risk factors that are associated with increased prevalence of these chronic diseases. Risk factors may or may not be amenable to modification, and the impact of their modification may not be certain (Table 8–2). Major risk factors in heart disease are high blood pressure, cigarette smoking, high levels of blood cholesterol, and overweight. These factors are modifiable, and reduced occurrence of heart disease is associated with their modification. Physical inactivity and stress have been shown to be associated with heart disease, and they could be modified, but the impact of their modification on the risk of acquiring heart disease is not entirely proven. Family history of heart disease is also important but obviously not modifiable; diabetes is an important factor, but the impact of its modification is not entirely certain.

The relationship between cigarette smoking and malignant neoplasms, especially respiratory cancers, has been proven inasmuch as current methodologies are capable of proving cause-and-effect relationships. Carcinogens at the work site are a major risk factor in cancers. Several studies have linked alcohol to some cancers, such as pancreatic cancer, and certain diets to colon cancers. Hypertension, smoking, and increased blood cholesterol are proven risk factors for stroke, while stress has been shown to be related to stroke, but the impact of its modification has not been shown. Accidents are associated with excessive alcohol use, excessive speed, and nonuse of seat belts. Smoking has been shown to be related to influenza and pneumonia, but its cessation, which logically should decrease the incidence of influenza and pneumonia, has not been confirmed to produce such a result.

Table 8–2 Major Causes of Death and Associated Risk Factors

Cause of Death	% of All Deaths	Associated Risk Factors		
		(1)	*(2)*	*(3)*
1. Heart disease	40	Hypertension Smoking Increased blood cholesterol Overweight	Physical inactivity Stress	Family history Diabetes
2. Malignant neoplasms	20	Smoking Worksite carcinogens	Alcohol Diet Environmental carcinogens	
3. Stroke	10	Hypertension Smoking Increased blood cholesterol	Stress	
4. Accidents	5	Alcohol Speed Seat belt nonuse		Drug abuse Medication use
5. Influenza and pneumonia	3		Smoking	

(1) Modifiable and of proven impact
(2) Modifiable, but impact is not entirely certain
(3) Modifiability and impact are not entirely certain

Source: Adapted from Figure 6, National Center for Health Statistics, *Health, United States, 1980,* U.S. Department of Health and Human Services publication no. (PHS) 81–1232 (Washington, D.C.: U.S. Government Printing Office, December 1980), and Table 5, V.J. Schoenbach, E.H. Wagner, and J.M. Karon, "The Use of Epidemiologic Data for Personal Risk Assessment in Health Hazard/Health Risk Appraisal Programs," *Journal of Chronic Disabilities* 36 (9): 625–638.

Risk factors associated with the prevalent chronic illnesses involve human behaviors and life styles of individuals. Increased blood cholesterol is related to eating food with large quantities of saturated fats, and overweight is related to overeating habits and lack of exercise. Smoking and alcohol use are centuries-old habits. Driving at high speeds, nonuse of seat belts, drug abuse, noncompliance with antihypertensive medication, physical inactivity, and not coping with stress represent various aspects of individual behaviors. Individual efforts are required to achieve the required changes in behaviors. The identification of hazardous life-style factors and the development of successful methods for achieving desired changes represent the domain of health promotion.

Health promotion and disease prevention activities may thus be classified into three broad areas:

1. Health promotion, which implies the changing of behaviors such as no longer smoking, decreasing the amount of saturated fats in the diet, or becoming physically active—activities that require individual efforts for sustained periods.
2. Health protection measures, which generally do not require individual efforts but involve changes at the community level. Examples include controlling carcinogens at the work site, controlling air pollution and hazardous waste disposal, and changing the ingredients of food products at the manufacturing source, as in the production of low-fat milk or low-calorie foods.
3. Preventive health services, which require minimal efforts on the part of the individual, such as visiting a health screening program for early case detection or a pediatrician's office to receive immunizations.

Many of the major causes of death are declining (Table 8–3). Between 1970 and 1980, for example, diseases of the heart declined 19%, stroke 37%, and motor vehicle accidents, 13%. Changes in the risk factors over time as a result of changes in human behavior have partially contributed to the decline in the deaths from these causes. On the other hand, malignant neoplasms—especially respiratory cancers—suicide, and homicide have increased rather drastically. This is especially the case between 1970 and 1980, compared with modest increases between 1950 and 1960, and 1960 and 1970. The increase in respiratory cancer is related to cigarette smoking and reflects an increase in lung cancer among women concomitant with increased smoking habits among them in recent years. Stress factors and social conditions may play an important role in suicide and homicide.

Table 8–3 Percentage of Change in Age-Adjusted Death Rates for Leading Causes of Death, United States, 1950–1980

Cause of Death	Percentage of Change 1950–60	Percentage of Change 1960–70	Percentage of Change 1970–80
Diseases of the heart	− 7.0	−11.4	−19.0
Malignant neoplasms	+ .3	+ 3.3	+ 3.3
Respiratory cancers	+50.0	+47.9	+29.2
Stroke	−10.2	−16.8	−37.4
Motor vehicle accidents	− 3.4	+21.8	−13.5
Suicide	− 3.6	+11.3	+ 3.4
Homicide	− 3.7	+75.0	+25.3

Source: Adapted from Tables 16–22, National Center for Health Statistics, *Health, United States, 1982*, U.S. Department of Health and Human Services publication no. (PHS) 81–1232 (Washington, D.C.: U.S. Government Printing Office, December 1982), 61–73.

The rise and fall in these causes of death seem concomitant with changes in human behaviors as well as changes in medical care.

CAUSES OF DEATH BY AGE GROUPS

Major causes of death for each age group are ranked in Table 8–4. The first two major causes of death in infants are prematurity- or birth-associated. Poor nutrition and maternal smoking are among the risk factors for bearing low birth weight infants. Detection of medical risks in advance of delivery and their management at delivery might help reduce birth-associated conditions. The first two causes of death in infants may thus be improved by proper and timely prenatal care. In the 10 years between 1970 and 1980, the percentage of white women receiving prenatal care in the first trimester increased from 72 to 79, and the corresponding percentages for black women were 44 and 69 (National Center for Health Statistics [NCHS] 1982). There is room for improvement in having more women participate in prenatal care, especially black women. Other causes of death in infants such as congenital birth defects and sudden infant deaths cannot be attributed to behavioral factors as far as known.

Table 8–4 Leading Causes of Death by Age Groups

Rank	Infants	1–14	15–24	25–64	65 and older
1	Prematurity-associated	Accidents other than MVA	Motor vehicle accidents	Heart disease	Heart disease
2	Birth-associated	Motor vehicle accidents	Accidents other than MVA	Cancer	Cancer
3	Congenital birth defects	Cancer	Suicide	Stroke	Stroke
4	Sudden infant deaths	Birth defects	Homicide	Cirrhosis of liver	Influenza and pneumonia
5	Influenza & pneumonia	Influenza & pneumonia	Cancer	Accidents other than MVA	Arterio-sclerosis

Source: Adapted from National Center for Health Statistics, *Health, United States, 1980,* U.S. Department of Health and Human Services publication no. (PHS) 81–1232 (Washington, D.C.: U.S. Government Printing Office, December 1980), 275–282.

The top two causes of death in children 1 to 14 years of age are accidents. Accidents other than motor vehicles include drownings, residential fires, and exposure to toxic substances and poisons. Deaths from non–motor vehicle accidents are higher (about one and a half times) for boys than for girls and about twice as high for black children as for white children (NCHS 1982). The opportunities for reducing the number of deaths among children due to these causes by changing behaviors are self-evident. Immunizations as preventive health services have played a key role in reducing or eliminating childhood diseases of measles, rubella, pertussis, polio, and mumps. Most children are immunized against most childhood diseases by the time they enter school (NCHS 1982). There are differences, however, by socioeconomic class, residence, and race.

In the age group of 15 to 24, the next major causes of death are suicide and homicide. Behavioral factors such as driving at high speeds, alcohol and drug use, coping with stress, and availability of guns contribute to these causes of death in this age group.

Heart disease, cancer, stroke, cirrhosis of the liver, and accidents are the five leading causes of death in persons 25 to 64 years of age. Risk factors described in Table 8–2 apply here. Heart disease, cancer, and stroke remain among the leading causes of death among persons 65 years of age and older. This is followed by influenza and pneumonia and arteriosclerosis. In addition to these causes of death, the elderly suffer from social isolation, depression, poor nutrition, and overmedication. Again, behavioral factors are crucial in alleviating the burden of illness among the elderly.

HEALTH PRACTICES AMONG AMERICANS

The National Health Interview Survey used a questionnaire in 1977 to collect data on the prevalence of seven presumably preventive-health practices among the noninstitutionalized U.S. population aged 20 years and older (NCHS November 4, 1980). The questions related to average number of hours of sleep, regularity of eating breakfast, frequency of eating snacks, level of physical activity, use of alcohol or tobacco, and body weight. It was found that about two-thirds of the population sleeps an average of 7 to 8 hours per night, with no substantial differences by demographic characteristics. It was reported that 50% of the population rated themselves at the same level of activity as others of the same age. Those who indicated that they were more active than others of the same age were more likely to be men than women, whites than blacks, and of higher than lower income.

Eating breakfast every day was reported by 58% of the population with differences noted among age and ethnic groups but not between the sexes. Eating snacks every day was reported by 38% of the population and was related to age of the respondent. It was also found that 30% of the population were above the desirable body weight; this was more so for women than men, blacks than whites, in the older than the younger age groups, and among the low- than the high-income groups.

Alcohol was reported in the form of occasional consumption by 42% of the population and was reported so by more women than men and young than old. Three or more drinks were reported by 14% of the population, and in this case it was more prevalent in men than women, whites than blacks, young than old, and high-income than low-income groups.

These health practices are the direct responsibility of the individual and fall in the class of health promotion activities. Their prevalence among the population generally and according to age, sex, and race groups provides baseline data against which subsequent changes can be measured and serves as a guide for focusing intervention procedures.

POLICY ON HEALTH PROMOTION AND DISEASE PREVENTION

The official publication of the U.S. Public Health Service (Public Health Reports 1983) puts forth a framework for a comprehensive national policy for health promotion and disease prevention. Three major areas of concerns were identified as follows:

1. Preventive health services. This category included high blood pressure control, family planning, pregnancy and infant health, immunization, and sexually transmitted disease control. An outline was given for each of these conditions as to the magnitude of the problem, effective procedures, and gaps in application or knowledge. For example, in high blood pressure control, the problem of differential access to health care by the various ethnic and racial groups and the adherence of most patients to prescribed medications remain an important goal. An estimated one-third of the 3.5 million births were unplanned, and more than 1 million pregnancies generally terminated legally. The poor, the black, and the teenager are the vulnerable groups for unintended pregnancy, unwanted birth, and abortion. Emphasis should be placed on prenatal care visits during the first trimester, especially by women who have a greater likelihood to deliver a low birth weight infant. The role of immunizations in the elimination or reduction of infectious diseases cannot be overemphasized.

2. Health protection. These activities include toxic agents and radiation control, occupational safety, accident prevention, fluoridation and dental health, and surveillance and control of infectious diseases. Toxic agents and radiation sources occur in industry as well as in medical and dental facilities and in agricultural products such as pesticides and herbicides. Occupational hazards may be con-

trolled by modifying the work place. However, exposure to carcinogens at the work site presents a more difficult problem. Occupational safety and accident prevention and control require a combination of changes on the part of the individual, the work place, and the home environment, as well as changes in legislation. Although the number of areas served by fluoridated water have increased tremendously, less than half of all Americans have access to fluoridated water. The problem is compounded by the fact that in areas where the water supply is not fluoridated, school drinking water is not fluoridated either. Infectious diseases continue to plague the population in spite of the fact that only pneumonia and influenza remain among the 10 leading causes of death in the United States. Surveillance and control efforts as well as development and use of new vaccines need to continue.

3. Health promotion. This class of activities includes smoking control, alcohol and drug abuse prevention, improved nutrition, physical fitness and exercise, and control of stress and violent behavior. Several millions have quit smoking since the 1964 publication of the *Surgeon General's Report on Smoking and Health*. This decline continues even for teenage smoking, especially among girls, for whom the smoking rate had been steadily increasing. It has been said that about 10% of all deaths in the United States are alcohol related. Legislation concerning alcohol use and driving had some effect on reducing deaths from motor vehicle accidents. Misuse of alcohol and other drugs, however, remains a major problem. A substantial proportion of the American population seem to have an inappropriate nutritional status insofar as about 15% of men and 25% of women are classified obese. Changes in nutritional practices, such as reducing saturated fat intake, are gaining popularity. Although benefits from physical fitness and exercise have not been completely studied, a larger proportion of the population have been engaged in improving their fitness by engaging in regular physical activity. The relationship between stress and physical disorders has been established, but the relationship between reducing the level of stress and lessening physical illness has not been fully assessed.

THE LIFETIME HEALTH-MONITORING PROGRAM

Preventive health services should be incorporated in medical care services and be paid either on a prepayment plan or fee for service as for other curative procedures (Breslow and Somers 1977). Preventive services should be offered according to the needs of specific age groups for whom the effectiveness of such services has already been established. The impact of the intervention procedure on the length and quality of life is an important parameter in determining the inclusion of a particular preventive procedure. Benefits, of course, must outweigh adverse effects.

The problem with this formulation is that often the epidemiologic evidence for effectiveness of a particular procedure is not always present, leaving the decision to professional judgment until further research is done. For example, a routine chest x-ray is no longer recommended for early detection of lung cancer, and a mammography, except for baseline information, is no longer required for women under age 50 for early detection of breast cancer. Often these preventive health services packages are sold to the community by health insurers and employers as a means for reducing the costs of medical care. This is difficult to document since it will take years before preventive services produce desired health states that in turn result in reduced costs of curative care.

HEALTH RISK APPRAISAL

Health risk appraisal is a technique designed to focus attention on risk factors and their consequences and is presumed to be an educational tool for motivating individuals to change their behaviors to more "healthful" patterns. Health risk appraisal is therefore an important aspect of health promotion and disease prevention programs.

An understanding of the methods used in arriving at a risk score and a critical appraisal of these methods and their implications are in order (Schoenbach, Wagner, and Karon 1983). First, risk probabilities for the leading causes of death are computed. These are personal characteristics and behaviors that have specified risk-of-death probabilities derived from epidemiologic and other data. For example, smoking one pack of cigarettes would have a risk factor value for lung cancer of 2. If there is more than one risk factor for a condition, the values of these factors form the basis for the derivation of a composite risk factor score. The risk factor or the composite risk factor values are multiplied by the average risk of death from a condition in individuals of the patient's age, race, and sex group in order to obtain a projected risk value. For a 40-year-old individual of a particular race and sex, the average risk of death from lung cancer might be 3 per 1,000. The projected risk for a similar individual who smokes one pack of cigarettes per day would be $2 \times 3 = 6$ (per 1,000).

This process is repeated for all diseases. Disease-specific projected risks are added to obtain an all-cause projected risk of death (Schoenbach, Wagner, and Karon 1983). For example, for a 40-year-old person who is obese, a smoker, inactive, a heavy user of alcohol, with elevated levels of blood pressure and cholesterol, the all-cause projected risk of death would be about 80 per 1,000 (6 for lung cancer, 36 for coronary heart disease, 5 for cirrhosis of the liver, and 33 for all other causes). The projected all-cause risk of death of 80 per 1,000 may be expressed, with the aid of appropriate tables, in the form of an *appraisal age*. The appraisal age is the age that corresponds to the projected all-cause risk of death of

80 per 1,000 for persons of the same race, sex, and age group of the individual. In the example cited, the appraisal age of the 40-year-old individual would be 45, which implies that the risk of death is higher than average. An appraisal age equal to the actual age would indicate that no risk is involved, and an appraisal age lower than the actual age would indicate a lower risk than average.

Finally, changing a particular behavior such as cessation of smoking would result in a theoretical reduction of the all-cause projected risk of death. This would be translated into a younger appraisal age, which would be a motivating force for the patient to change behavior accordingly.

There are at least five limitations with the health risk appraisal techniques and their applications (Schoenbach, Wagner, and Karon 1983)

1. There are considerable variations in mortality among geographic groups, and several measurement errors are inherent in the quantification of a particular characteristic as well as in the specificity of the cause of death as listed on the death certificate. These variations and errors would lead to a risk assessment that may not be accurate.

2. The method of computation of the risk factor value is made in reference to the average risk of 1.0 instead of the actual risk of those without the particular behavior. For example, the role of cigarette smoking in the development of coronary heart disease would have a risk factor value of 1.5, using the average risk of 1.0 for the particular age-race-sex group. Non-smokers, however, may be assigned a risk factor of 0.4; if that were used instead of the average risk factor of 1.0, the risk factor value for those who smoke would become 3.8 (1.5 ÷ 0.4) rather than 1.5 (Schoenbach, Wagner, and Karon 1983). This would indicate that the risk computed for the health risk appraisal score is an underestimate of the actual risk.

3. The method of computation of the composite risk factor value may also be questioned. In the so-called credit-debit system, the amounts by which risk factors exceed the average of 1.0 are added, and the risk factor values that are less than 1.0 are multiplied and their product is added to the former quantity (Schoenbach, Wagner, and Karon 1983). A composite risk factor computed for arteriosclerotic heart disease in a 40-year-old person who possesses the known risk factors would be 2.7. A multiplicative procedure in which the individual risk factor values are multiplied to obtain the composite risk factor would result in an amount of 1.4 instead of 2.7. Because of the possible confounding effects of various factors, it cannot be assumed that risk factors act independently of one another. Indeed many work together in a synergistic fashion. This possibility makes a multiple logistic function method preferable in computing the composite risk factors that either the credit-debit or the multiplicative method (Schoenbach, Wagner, and Karon 1983).

4. Competing risks are ignored in deriving the all-cause mortality risk (Schoenbach, Wagner, and Karon 1983). Competing risks mean that when a person's risk of dying from a particular disease is increased, the risk of dying from a second disease would have to be lower than the actual risk of dying computed on the basis of the singular presence of the second disease. Health risk appraisal computations do not take this into account.
5. Lumping causes of death, other than the leading causes of death, into one group could produce distorted estimates of risk for the individual in question.

In spite of these limitations, health risk appraisal is becoming a popular tool for motivating individuals to change their life styles. Refinements of the methods are desirable so that more accurate estimates are obtained. Not promising youth and longevity but making honest presentations and inferences would not represent misuse of this innovation.

POLICY DESPITE UNCERTAINTIES ABOUT CAUSE AND EFFECT

The causal connection of many behavioral factors to disease remains to be proven. The role of physical activity in health is yet to be clearly documented. Jogging, for example, is one means of achieving physical fitness. Issues raised about jogging include the acute or immediate hazards; delayed or long-term effect; the favorable, adverse, or no effect on health; and the nature of the public health stand on its practice (Ibrahim 1983). Although all the evidence is not yet in, the conclusion of beneficial effects "is substantiated by the consistency of the findings, the clear effect of exercise on physical fitness, and a plausible mechanism and process by which physical exercise protects against morbidity and mortality from cardiovascular diseases" (p. 136). Since the epidemiologic data "tips the balance in favor of promoting physical activity" (p. 137); since the harmful effects, although not unimportant, could be eliminated by proper means; and since the public interest in physical exercise is so great, it would seem that "the public health stand should take the form of encouragement or even advocacy of physical exercise by the American public" (p. 137).

The association between cigarette smoking and lung cancer, heart disease, and other conditions is so conclusive that cigarette smoking must be considered as one of the causes of these disorders. The precise nature and degree by which smoking could be linked to lung cancer or heart disease cannot be determined; experimental proof will not be forthcoming, and new observational studies cannot enlighten us much more (Ibrahim 1976). The promotion of antismoking campaigns is an indispensable pillar in any health promotion and disease prevention programs despite the absence of a conclusive proof as to cause-and-effect relationships.

The regulation of environmental containments in the absence of precise scientific data creates a major dilemma. Decisions such as banning saccharin or making drinking water "safe" are made before obtaining adequate scientific estimation of public health risk (Ibrahim and Christman 1977). In these and other areas where health protection measures are needed, strong scientific risk estimates are in short supply. Policy must nevertheless be made while more research is being undertaken.

The preceding account emphasizes the role of judgment in policy. There are those, of course, who want to wait for the "last human clinical trial to be completed before making recommendations for public use" and those who want to push "beyond the margin of scientific reason" in recommending certain behaviors (McGinnis 1981, p. 26). As health promotion and disease prevention policies are made and programs are implemented, several safeguards must be observed (McGinnis 1981). Programs designed to change behaviors must not use or be perceived to use elements of coercion. Health promotion is not a panacea, and changing individual behaviors will not result in achieving complete health. Environmental factors and biologic susceptibility contribute greatly to the health of populations. Finally, one must avoid the emergence of the "healthy elite"—the highly educated person of high economic means who is not obese and who does not smoke or drink—at the expense of a large segment of the population at high risk of illness and in need of attention.

SOME PARADOXES

A combination of attitudes on the part of the medical profession, the public, financiers of medical research and education, insurance companies, and funding agencies of medical research has resulted in a system of "sickness" care rather than "health" care (Yankauer 1983). In addition, the unique mix of private and public delivery and financing of services has tipped the balance toward the provision of medical care and forced preventive health services to occupy a distant second place. The problem is compounded by several paradoxes: the practice of preventive measures in the context of only periodic examinations rather than regular routine physician visits, the practice by physicians of nonrecommended preventive procedures versus the nonpractice of recommended procedures, state laws requiring immunization of school children versus laws not requiring passive protective devices in cars, and requirements of family planning clinics to inform parents of teenagers about their pregnancies but independent rights to a week-old fetus (Yankauer 1983).

The monetary rewards, profits, and political influence of special interest groups could explain many of these paradoxes. Regardless of the reasons, the mix of private and public concerns, which could work to the detriment of the provision of preventive health services, needs to be considered in the formulation of policy. Physicians in private practice should run their own practices the best way they know and individualize their care according to the needs of each patient. However, when public funds are involved either by paying for services delivered by the private sector, or by directly providing government services, only proven preventive health care procedures should be considered acceptable (more on these issues in Chapter 9).

CONCLUSION

Health promotion and disease prevention (hp/dp) may be viewed within the context of the changing nature of the leading causes of death and illness. Health promotion implying changes in behaviors, health protection involving community and environmental changes, and preventive services meaning early diagnosis and immunizations are three broad classes that constitute hp/dp.

The prevalence of health behaviors in the population generally and in age-race-sex specific groups provides baseline data against which subsequent changes can be noted.

A comprehensive national policy for health promotion and disease prevention has been proposed by the Public Health Service. It includes detailed objectives, services, and desired changes in the three areas of promotion, protection, and preventive services.

Health risk appraisal is a technique intended to draw attention to risk factors and their consequences. It is a useful educational tool but needs extensive refinements before its purpose is properly realized.

BIBLIOGRAPHY

Breslow L, Somers AR: The lifetime Health-Monitoring Program. *N Eng J Med* 1977; 296(11): 601–608.

Ibrahim MA: The cigarette smoking/lung cancer hypothesis, editorial. *Amer J Pub Health* 1976; 66(2): 132–133.

Ibrahim MA: In support of jogging, editorial. *Amer J Pub Health* 1983; 73(2): 136–137.

Ibrahim MA, Christman RF: Drinking water and carcinogenesis: The dilemmas, editorial. *Amer J Pub Health* 1977; 67(8): 719–720.

McGinnis JM: The future and healthy people: Political and social implications. *Mobius 1981*. Regents of the University of California, 1981, pp 18–28.

National Center for Health Statistics. Health practices among adults: United States 1977. *Advance Data*, 64; 1–9, November 4, 1980.

National Center for Health Statistics: *Health, United States, 1980.* US Dept of Health and Human Services publication No. (PHS) 81–1232. Government Printing Office, December 1980.

National Center for Health Statistics: *Health, United States, 1982.* US Dept of Health and Human Services publication No. (PHS) 83–1232. Government Printing Office, December 1982.

Schoenbach VJ, Wagner EH, Karon JM: The use of epidemiologic data for personal risk assessment in Health Hazard/Health Risk Appraisal Programs. *J Chron Dis* 1983; 36(9): 625–638.

Yankauer A: Public and private prevention, editorial. *Amer J Pub Health* 1983; (9): 1032–1034.

U.S. Department of Health and Human Services: Public health service implementation plans for attaining the objectives for the nation. *Public Health Reports* 1983; Sept.-Oct.

Chapter 9

Health Screening and Periodic Examinations

Your body is a wonderful machine. You own and operate it. You can't buy new lungs and heart when your own are worn out. Let a doctor overhaul you once a year.

Haven Emerson

Health screening refers to the application of various tests to apparently healthy individuals to sort out those who probably have risk factors or are in the early stages of specified conditions. These individuals are then subjected to a battery of tests, procedures, and medical examinations to confirm or refute the findings of the health screening procedure. Conventional health screening is usually conducted outside the physician's office. Periodic medical examinations are similar in concept to health screening except that they are performed in a physician's office and may consist of more sophisticated tests such as an electrocardiogram, as well as a physical examination. Health screening and periodic examinations belong to the class of preventive health services, which together with health protection and health promotion activities form what has been referred to as health promotion and disease prevention described in Chapter 8. Preventive health services represent a special set of long-standing activities that are addressed separately in this section.

Emphasis on preventive health services began at the turn of the century. The discovery of low physical fitness and potentially correctable defects among military recruits encouraged health professionals to advance periodic health examinations as a method for uncovering and correcting these problems. The very successful well-baby clinics and school health programs provided a model for preventive exams for adults, which were introduced by insurance companies in 1909 (Yankauer 1981). Physicians as well as the public have endorsed and engaged in health screening and periodic examination activities for a long time with little questioning of their ultimate value.

In the 1960s and beyond, as a result of the public's sophistication, introduction and application of rigorous research methods, and increased medical costs due to the application of advanced technologies, the benefits as well as potential harmful effects of preventive health services have become subjects for careful scrutiny. Another important aspect of the application of preventive health services is their potential incorporation into regular ambulatory visits to a physician instead of a community setting. Targeting preventive health services to populations at high risk is another important consideration by those responsible for the provision of health care.

SOME BASIC PRINCIPLES

Criteria for the Condition

Certain criteria must be met before deciding on a policy for screening for a particular condition. The condition must represent an important health problem as to the magnitude of mortality, incidence, and prevalence of the condition itself and its consequences. The condition should have a preclinical or an asymptomatic period that is identifiable by a test or a maneuver and should be amenable to intervention at this phase of its course. It is further assumed that intervention at this stage would lengthen or improve the quality of life more than intervention when the condition becomes symptomatic and recognizable during a physician visit.

Without experimental evidence it is conceivable that lengthening of life may be apparent only as a result of selecting a starting point for measuring survival after detecting the "early stage" of the disease (Sackett 1980). The five-year survival among patients who have been diagnosed (and treated earlier) may appear to be better by one year, for example, than those who were not diagnosed until they experienced symptoms that brought them to medical care for proper treatment. It is conceivable in this case that the five-year survival measurement was made one year earlier from the usual time of diagnosis. That is, the patients have been detected one year earlier, giving them "an extra year of disease" rather than an "extra year of life" (Sackett 1980).

Detection of a risk factor or an early stage of a disease in an otherwise normal individual may also have consequences as a result of "labeling" the individual as being at risk or having an early stage of a disease. Consequences may include absenteeism from work or school, psychosocial manifestations such as anxiety, depression, and unnecessary restriction of social or physical activities. Untoward effects of labeling must obviously be weighed against beneficial effects of the early detection. Conversely labeling a sick individual as having a "clean bill of health" as a result of the application of a set of screening procedures may be equally damaging. Such a person may overestimate the real value of health screening and thus may proceed to indulge in potentially harmful life-style behaviors.

Criteria for Test or Maneuver

Screening tests, especially when applied to large masses of populations, should be simple, safe, acceptable, and administered at a reasonable cost. Advances in technologies have played a major role in this regard. These advances, however, led to the application of many more tests than known to physicians to be of demonstrable value. Because 12 tests could be performed for the price of 2, the inclination is to perform the 12. Two questions may be raised with regard to performing too many tests: What should be done with a test result for which no known intervention is available? And what is the social and physical impact on the individual of finding something wrong simply as a function of doing more tests? The percentage of normal people with at least one abnormal test result increases from 5% when 1 test is performed, to 23% when 5 are performed, to 65% when 20 are performed, and to 99% when 100 tests are performed (Sackett 1978).

A screening test has several properties that must be understood and evaluated before a policy decision is made as to its inclusion in or exclusion from a health screening program. The important properties are sensitivity, specificity, and predictive value (Table 9–1). Sensitivity refers to the percentage of individuals who met the test criterion for being positive among those who clearly have the disease. Specificity refers to the percentage of individuals who satisfied the test criterion for being negative among those individuals in whom the disease is clearly absent. Predictive value of a test refers to the proportion of individuals who have been found clearly to have the disease among those who satisfied the test criterion for being positive. Ideally one would like to approach 100% for all of these properties, but since they are interrelated, a change in the value of one property usually occurs at the expense of the other. Some judgment needs to be made with regard to the property that, depending on the question being asked, would be more crucial than others.

Specificity may be measured as described in the previous paragraph, that is, the percentage of true negatives among individuals in whom the disease is clearly absent, or by taking advantage of the fact that specificity relates to the bulk of individuals (those who do not have the disease). The false positives (individuals positive on the test but in whom the disease was found absent after further diagnostic investigations) may be used as the numerator to be divided by the total number of individuals involved (T), resulting in a quotient that is essentially the nonspecificity of the test. Specificity then may be calculated by simply subtracting this quantity from 1.

Predictive value of a test is perhaps the most important property insofar as health service research and policy making are concerned. If the predictive value is

Table 9–1 Sensitivity, Specificity, and Predictive Value of a Screening Test

| Test Criterion | Disease | | Total |
	Clearly Present	Clearly Absent	
Positive	True positives	False positives	t_3
Negative	False negatives	True negatives	t_4
Total	t_1	t_2	T

$$\text{Sensitivity} = \frac{\text{true positives}}{t_1} \times 100$$

$$\text{Specificity} = \frac{\text{true negatives}}{t_2} \times 100$$

$$\text{Predictive value} = \frac{\text{true positives}}{t_3} \times 100$$

small—that is, a small proportion of the bulk of those who met the positive test criterion (t_3) is found to have the disease after elaborate testing—it follows that considerable resources would have to be used in order to separate the false positives. It is here that consideration must be made about balancing resources available with the potential harmful effects resulting from not identifying a particular case.

Predictive value is influenced by the sensitivity and specificity of the test and the prevalence of the condition of interest. As the prevalence of the condition ($t_1 \div T$), increases so would the predictive value of the test. The predictive value would also increase when the sensitivity and specificity of the test increase. This relationship may be used in recommending the test for high-risk groups, in whom the prevalence of the condition would be higher than the total population, as a means of increasing its yield or predictive value. This approach would lead to better use of available resources, thereby reduction of medical care costs.

Criteria for the Intervention Procedure or Program

An intervention procedure must be available, accessible, and acceptable to the population for which it applies. The procedure must be an integral part of or easily linked to an existing medical care system. The procedure or program must be of proven efficacy and effectiveness, preferably on the basis of the results of randomized clinical or community controlled trials. In the absence of randomized trials, evidence from observational studies must be of high quality. Finally, the intervention procedure or program must be administered effectively with available resources.

SCIENTIFIC EVIDENCE FOR EFFICACY AND EFFECTIVENESS

The value of performing periodic medical examinations at all or at certain intervals (usually annual), as well as the content of such examinations, has been questioned. The worth of several tests and procedures has often lacked sound scientific basis. Self-selection may partially explain the presumed benefits of periodic health examinations in that healthy or health-conscious individuals are the ones who seek periodic examinations. Few randomized trials have been conducted in an effort to answer some of these questions.

Annual multiphasic health checkups were evaluated by a randomized controlled trial on 10,000 men and women aged 35 to 54 who have been subscribers in the Kaiser Foundation Health Plan (Dales, Friedman, and Collen 1979). The checkups consisted of completion of a medical questionnaire and a physical examination; performance of several tests and procedures such as EKG determination; assessment of blood pressure, vision, hearing, and eye tension tests; and analysis of urine and blood. Pap smears were done on all women, mammography on women older than 48 years of age, and sigmoidoscopy on all persons older than 40 years of age. End results of this trial consisted of clinical and hospital use, self-reported disability, and mortality.

No statistically significant differences were revealed when patients who were urged to participate in the multiphasic health checkups were compared with those who were not. However, comparison of population subsegments in those who participated with those who did not revealed (1) decreased self-reported disability in men 45 to 54 years of age and (2) fewer deaths from hypertension and colorectal cancer. These findings bear added significance when considered with concomitant and relevant changes that provided possible mechanisms for achieving end results. These changes consisted of increases in the identification and control of individuals with high blood pressure and high blood cholesterol and those who were diabetic, obese, and smokers. In addition, early diagnosed colorectal cancer was found in the group who participated in the periodic health checkups. These findings highlighted the importance of targeting preventive health services as evident from the review of the comprehensive and systematic approach used by the Canadian Task Force on Health Examinations.

The Canadian Task Force on Periodic Health Examinations

The task force critically appraised periodic health examinations on several grounds ("The Periodic Health Examination" 1979). It noted that the content of these examinations consisted of many tests and procedures with no or little evidence of worth. There was no solid basis for performance of the examinations at yearly intervals, and indeed many of its components could be performed at much longer intervals. Finally, the population engaged in this practice is usually that of the upper economic classes and of certain age and sex groups: individuals who are not necessarily at the greatest risk or need.

The Canadian task force developed several criteria as the basis for making its recommendations. The criteria covered three main areas: those that are related to the quality of the scientific evidence, those that are related to the burden of suffering, and those that are related to the characteristics of the intervention procedures or tests.

The quality of evidence was ranked from good (I) to poor (III) as follows:

I. good evidence that is supported by at least one properly conducted randomized controlled trial
II. fair evidence
   a. evidence that is based on more than one well-designed case-control or cohort study
   b. evidence that is based on the results of analysis of temporal or geographic trends
III. poor evidence that is based on opinions of respected authorities and expert committees

The second criterion was the burden of suffering resulting from the condition for which a test or procedure is being performed. The social, emotional, physical, and economic impact of a condition on the individual, family, and society formed the basis for judging the degree of the burden of an illness. The burden was judged according to these factors as substantial, equivocal, or not substantial.

Characteristics of intervention procedures or tests formed the third criterion. Potential risks and benefits of a particular procedure or test were important considerations. The sensitivity, specificity, and predictive value were entered into the judgment equation as well. Finally, and of equal importance, were the safety, simplicity, cost, and acceptability of the test or procedure.

These criteria were used in the formulation of a recommendation that may be viewed as a continuum extending from inclusion to exclusion of a test or procedure in a set of activities that comprise a periodic health examination. These recommendations may be summarized as follows:

- The criteria were fully met to justify the inclusion of a test or procedure, as for blood pressure measurements, immunizations, and mammography for early detection of breast cancer in women over 50.
- The criteria were fairly met to justify the inclusion of a test or procedure, as for Pap smear for early detection of cervical cancer, especially in high-risk individuals.
- The criteria were poorly met. Judgment must be used for the inclusion or exclusion of a particular test or procedure. An example of this class is testing the eye tension for early detection of primary open-angle glaucoma.
- The criteria were fairly unmet, therefore justifying the possible exclusion of a particular test or procedure. Chest x-ray and sputum cytology for early detection of lung cancer are examples of this class.
- The criteria were substantially unmet, therefore justifying the exclusion of a particular test or procedure as in the case of testing the entire population for tuberculosis.

On the basis of this strategy the task force recommended that a routine annual checkup be abandoned in favor of a selective approach based on the condition, as well as the age and sex, of the individual.

This selective approach forms the basis of a policy that is proposed to provide a lifetime plan of preventive health services. It is further recommended that case finding should be performed during a routine medical care visit and not by door-to-door screening. Such an approach is quite reasonable since a substantial proportion of the population see a physician once a year, and a vast majority see a physician within three years. However, pregnant women, the very young, and the very old must receive adequate preventive services regardless of routine physician visits. Finally, the task force recommended research in areas where firm recommendations could not be made.

The American Cancer Society Recommendations

The American Cancer Society report on the cancer-related health checkup (1980) included recommendations for the early detection of cancer in asymptomatic persons. Chest x-ray, for example, was recommended annually for early detection of lung cancer in high-risk persons. It is not recommended according to revised criteria. Sigmoidoscopy, which was recommended annually for persons more than 40 years of age, is recommended for persons more than 50 years of age, every three to five years after two negative exams one year apart. Pap smear is recommended for women 20 to 65 years of age, and for those under 20 if sexually active, at a frequency of every three years after two negative exams one year apart. More frequent testing is recommended in high-risk women. The previous recommendation of annual pelvic and breast physical examinations has been extended to three years in women 20 to 40 and every year in women who are older than 40. Mammography is recommended once for baseline information on women 35 to 40 years of age and annually for those who are older than 50.

The American Cancer Society should be congratulated for revising its recommendations and extending the interval between tests. Even with these revisions the cost for heeding these recommendations is enormous. The cost of prevention must, however, be compared with the cost of treatment after the diagnosis has been made and the consequent loss of human life.

CASE EXAMPLES

Congenital Disease of the Hip

Neonatal screening for this condition has been based on the premise that an application of a simple clinical test to neonates would lead to an early diagnosis of congenital disease of the hip, which when treated at that time would result in more improved functioning than when treated after the patient develops symptoms. The characteristics of the clinical test and its application to neonates as well as the potential end results have been tested against criteria that formed the basis of recommending or not recommending such a procedure (Parkin 1981).

No randomized controlled trials have provided satisfactory evidence for the benefits to be accrued from neonatal screening for congenital disease of the hip. Since the birth prevalence of abnormal hips is greater than that of subsequent manifest disease as a result of spontaneous recovery, misleading statements about the efficacy of the test could be made. Since the number of false positives is large, meaning low predictive value for a positive test, the use of medical resources in making a definitive diagnosis may be questioned. The test has no reliable data on sensitivity, specificity, or predictive values. In the light of these uncertainties it may be concluded that mass screening for dislocation of the hip is unwarranted since it does not meet the standard criteria for recommending screening (Parkin 1981; Frankenburg 1981).

A distinction must be made between the performance of mass screening that would be publicly financed and performance of various tests and procedures by physicians in their practices. As stated, private practice must be left to the discretion of the physician and the patient. Three rather simple questions may guide decisions with regard to screening: ''What good may it do? What harm may it do? What harm may be done by not doing it?'' (Illingworth 1971).

Cervical Cancer

There is general agreement, albeit without experimental evidence, that screening for cervical cancer by Pap smears would result in reduction of mortality from invasive cancer as a consequence of early detection and treatment. The observational evidence consisted of an association between decreased mortality from cervical cancer in populations where screening tests have been performed. In addition, the rate of clinical cancer decreases as the rate of screening of women at risk increases. The problem of these observational studies is that they do not provide firm evidence of the effectiveness of screening programs. For example, it is not known precisely what proportion of cervical lesions in the preinvasive stage progressed to the invasive stage. In addition, a decline in mortality has been observed in areas where screening for cervical cancer was not performed, except that the decline is not as great as in areas where screening has been performed.

Nevertheless, the procedure is of some demonstrable benefit and is acceptable to the majority of the population. Randomized controlled trials will not be performed because of ethical and technical reasons. Therefore the procedure is recommended, but several issues need to be addressed: the frequency of performing the screening test, the cost effectiveness of the procedure, and its potential adverse physical or psychological effects (Ibrahim 1978).

With regard to the frequency of Pap smear screening, the recommendations of the American Cancer Society and the American College of Obstetrics and Gynecology are at odds ("Pap Smear Controversy" 1981). The American Cancer Society position is that for most women a Pap test at three-year intervals would be just as productive for detecting tumors before the invasive stage as the annual test and "three times as cost effective." This recommendation is modified in that it should be performed after two negative annual tests, and the interval may be shortened in high-risk groups. The American College of Obstetrics and Gynecology position is that extending the interval between tests would mean that some lesions would go undetected in their earlier stage and therefore proceed to an invasive stage. Lengthening the interval would therefore result in "trading dollars for lives."

The American Cancer Society offers criteria of screening but takes advantage of the special needs of age-specific and special risk groups. The college recommends that extending the interval should be a matter between patients and their physicians. The society further believes that preinvasive cancer precedes the invasive stage by about 30 years, and therefore lengthening the interval of screening would still allow for the detection of the disease and also would reduce the risk of treating tumors that do not need treatment. This is especially the case since some cases are diagnosed erroneously, and some retrogress naturally. The society refers to the savings if the interval is extended and points to other countries such as Britain and Canada that have lengthened their interval to three or five years.

The college counteracts the society's claims by indicating that the reduction noted in cancer mortality has been associated with annual screening procedures and not procedures that extended three years. Further, it is claimed that the time between the preinvasive stage and the invasive stage may not be as long as reported. The college further states that the test is inexpensive and should be made accessible to poor and minority populations, that there are no definable high-risk groups since most women must be considered at high risk, and finally that the one year is a convenient bench mark. The society and the college are using the same data to arrive at two different conclusions. Both groups are trying to make policy recommendations on the basis of available evidence—a commendable behavior provided that neither group deliberately misuses the information.

Breast Cancer

Some believe that early detection of breast cancer has not been useful in reducing mortality from this condition. This conclusion is based on the fact that age-specific death rates from breast cancer in the United States have not changed over the last several years. However, the stability of mortality over time does not necessarily negate the potential benefit of screening programs. It is conceivable that the incidence of breast cancer is increasing, and this coupled with improved survival as a result of early detection could result in no change in death rates. Furthermore, increased survival may not necessarily be attributable to early diagnosis of the disease but may be an apparent increase due to women living longer, knowing that they have breast cancer, rather than actually gaining extra years of life (Sackett 1980).

A randomized controlled trial was conducted on 31,000 women who were offered mammography and clinical examinations at least once a year and 31,000 women who were offered the procedures only on their request (Shapiro 1979). These patients were subscribers to the Health Insurance Plan of Greater New York (HIP). After three and one-half years of follow-up it was shown that the percentage of patients with breast cancer in whom there was no evidence of cancer spread was higher in the screened group than in the control group. Furthermore, the case fatality rate was twice as high in the control group (33%) as the screened group. Further analysis showed that mammography had its most benefit in women older than 50, and it may not be effective and in fact may be even hazardous in women younger than 50.

The American Cancer Society recommendations with regard to mammography are to obtain baseline measure in women between the ages of 35 and 40, to consult a physician as to the advisability of performing mammography in women younger than age 50, and to perform the procedure annually in women older than 50. The scientific evidence underpinning this recommendation is firm and quite persuasive.

CONCLUSION

Physicians and the general population have endorsed the concepts and activities of health screening and periodic health examinations for a long time without critical questioning of their ultimate value.

Criteria for the disease, test, and intervention program have been carefully formulated. The Canadian Task Force on Periodic Health Examinations ranked the quality of evidence and used the rankings, in addition to the degree of burden of illness and characteristics of the procedure, as the basis for making action recommendations.

Screening for congenital disease of the hip, preinvasive cervical cancer, and breast cancer is appraised against available scientific evidence. Policies for health screening and periodic examinations are critically examined and frequently updated.

BIBLIOGRAPHY

American Cancer Society report on the cancer-related health checkup 1980; *CA* 30(4): 194–240.

Dales LG, Friedman GD, Collen MF: Evaluating periodic multiphasic health checkups: A controlled trial. *J Chron Dis* 1979; 32: 385–404.

Emerson H: The protection of health through periodic medical examinations (1922), in Selected Papers of Haven Emerson 1949. Battle Creek; W.K. Kellogg Foundation. Cited in Yankauer A: The ups and downs of prevention. *Am J Public Health* 1981; 71(1): 6–9.

Frankenburg WK: To screen or not to screen: Congenital dislocation of the hip, editorial. *Am J Pub Health* 1981; 71(12): 1311–1313.

Ibrahim MA: The case for cervical cancer screening, editorial. *Amer J Pub Health* 1978; 68: 114–115.

Illingworth RS: Discussion of diagnostic catheter examinations of the newborn by Norman T. Quinn. *Clin Ped 1971;* 10: 254.

Pap smear controversy pits cancer society vs ob-gyns. *Hospital Practice*, February 1981, pp 16, 21, 24, 29.

Parkin DM : How successful is screening for congenital disease of the hip? *Amer J Pub Health* 1981; 71(12): 1378–1383.

The periodic health examination. Task force report. *Canad Med Assoc J* 1979; 121: 1195–1254.

Sackett DL: Clinical diagnosis and the clinical laboratory. *Clinical Investigation Medicine* 1978; 1: 37–43.

Sackett DL: Evaluation of health service, in Last JM (ed): *Public Health and Preventive Medicine.* New York, Appleton-Century-Crofts, 1980.

Shapiro S: Evidence on screening for breast cancer from a randomized trial. *Cancer* 1979; 39: 2772–2782.

Yankauer A: The ups and downs of prevention. *Am J Public Health* 1981; 71(1): 6–9.

Part IV

Procedures and Personnel

Chapter 10

Technologies: Coronary Artery Bypass and Computed Tomography

As the popularity and attractiveness of sophisticated advanced technology increase, so do questions on costs, safety, and efficacy. The central question is, Does the benefit outweigh the cost? Government attention was specifically drawn to this issue in 1975 in reference to medical services to be reimbursed from Medicare and Medicaid programs (Banta 1982). It was noted that "Medicare does not finance or engage in biomedical research. It does, however, finance the results of this research" (Gaus 1982, p. 6). The interest in technology by Congress was highlighted by establishing a National Center for Health Care Technology in 1978, a center that disappeared in 1981 as the result of budget cuts.

Although the United States is not alone in facing the issues surrounding the use of expensive technologies, other western countries may be somewhat ahead of the United States (Russell 1982). The regionalization of health services in Sweden is an example of increased emphasis on primary care coupled with the efficient use of hospital facilities and sophisticated technologies. The national health service of Great Britain exercises considerable care in selecting procedures that have proven beneficial and therefore provides an acceptable rationale for the use and allocation of limited resources. France developed a system to discourage the widespread use of technology by employing rigid criteria such as an equipment-population ratio in the allocation of specific resources.

Changes over time in the use of hospital tests and procedures have been analyzed. In one study 1,203 patients were hospitalized in either of two periods, 1972 or 1977, for 10 diagnoses (Showstack, Schroeder, and Matsumoto 1982). The total number of tests and procedures, controlling for the length of hospital stay and severity of condition, remained generally unchanged. However, certain new diagnostic procedures were significantly increased. Of special interest from an epidemiologic perspective, however, is the discharge status as expressed in percentage of dead, which did not change in spite of the increased use of sophisticated tests and procedures (Table 10–1).

Table 10–1 Use of Selected Technologies and Discharge Status in Two Time Periods

Diagnosis	(1) 1972	1977	(2) 1972	1977	(3) 1972	1977
Acute myocardial infarction	3	32	0.5	2.3	15	13
Lung cancer	0	15	0.9	1.2	22	24
Respiratory distress syndrome	0	24	2.3	8.2	15	18
Kidney transplantation	2	20	—	—	5	5

(1) Ultrasound or echo cardiography—percentage of patients using service. All differences between the two periods are statistically significant.

(2) Nuclear medicine—adjusted mean times of use. Differences between the two periods, except for lung cancer, are statistically significant.

(3) Discharge status—percentage dead. All differences between the two periods are *not* statistically significant.

Source: Adapted from Tables 2 and 5, J.A. Showstack, S.A. Schroeder, and M.F. Matsumoto, "Changes in the Use of Medical Technologies, 1972–77. A Study of 10 Inpatient Diagnoses," *New England Journal of Medicine* 1982 (306): 706–712.

The considerable appeal of technologies does not seem to be lessening. The major problem with them is that they are introduced prematurely before the benefits and hazards are assessed properly and before adequate evaluation using rigorous methods such as the randomized controlled trial is undertaken. The result is an ethical dilemma as the presumed benefits of the device or procedure preclude the use of randomized controlled trials in which a control group would be denied access to and use of the technology being tested. This would leave only observational studies as an acceptable method of evaluation, which often produce inconclusive findings. Three courses of action may be offered to remedy the situation partially (Gaus 1982, p. 7):

1. assessment of medical practice in its entirety since "many current medical practices (such as multiphasic screening) are done as a matter of course with no hard evidence to support their efficacy or efficiency"
2. evaluation of new procedures before the adoption and diffusion of such procedures
3. assessment of potential benefits of proposed major procedures *before* allocating funds for relevant medical research.

CORONARY ARTERY BYPASS (CAB)

The concept of increasing the blood supply to the heart muscle in spite of clogged coronary arteries has been in existence for some time (Harrison 1981).

Increasing the vascularization of the heart muscle by manipulation as well as the insertion of irritants at the origins of the coronary arteries began in the late 1930s. The next development was to implant one of the internal mammary arteries in a tunnel cut in the heart muscle in the belief that such a healthy artery would stimulate the formation of small blood vessels, which in turn would provide the necessary blood circulation. In the late 1960s a piece of the saphenous vein was used to connect the aorta to the coronary vessels beyond the obstructed segment. By 1968 the technologies of saphenous vein bypass surgery were fully developed and used widely. There are those who prefer the use of the internal mammary arteries, instead of a piece of the saphenous vein, to provide the necessary blood supply by connecting the artery to the segment of a coronary artery beyond the obstruction.

Methodologic Issues

Several issues should be considered in the evaluation of coronary artery bypass. First is the issue of prolonging survival versus improving the quality of life. Having both outcomes would, of course, be ideal, but having one or the other offers the opportunity to argue for or against the procedure. The second important issue is the definition of a case and the type of disease for which the operation would be most beneficial. Criteria for inclusion in or exclusion from a study population are crucial in order to arrive at the proper conclusion. Distinctions must be made between stable and unstable angina; one-, two-, or three-vessel disease; and poor or adequate functional status of the heart muscle (primarily the left ventricle).

The use of randomized trials is, of course, the best method to evaluate coronary artery bypass. Observational studies with their inherent problems, discussed previously, have special problems in reference to coronary artery bypass. Two important confounding factors complicate observational studies, especially those extending over a long period. In addition to variability among institutions, operative mortality is declining over time because of improved methods and procedures of surgery. Improved operative mortality and indeed medical treatment as well add to the complexity of making correct inferences with regard to the efficacy of surgery when compared with medical treatment using observational methods of investigation. In the 1970s, the superiority of medical treatment over bypass surgery may have been confounded by high operative mortality rates. In the 1980s, superiority of surgery over medical treatment may have been confounded by the improved operative mortality rates.

Another problem in comparing medical and surgical treatments is that of crossovers of cases (Chalmers et al. 1978). These crossovers are cases that have been assigned to the medical group but later underwent surgery and cases assigned to the surgical group on whom the surgery was not performed. The following four approaches may be considered:

1. Analyze according to the original assignment, keeping the cases in the original groups as if no switching has occurred.
2. Analyze according to actual treatment received; that is, rearrange the categories.
3. Analyze according to the original assignment but delete those who switched.
4. Analyze according to the original assigned group but consider those who switched as lost to follow-up in the application of life table analysis.

Each of these analyses answers a different question. Some recommend that analysis should be carried out according to all four approaches to detect consistency in the results.

A Randomized Trial

In 1977 the results of the randomized Veterans Administration Cooperative Study in the treatment of chronic stable angina was published (Murphy et al. 1977). All male patients with chronic stable angina entering any one of 14 participating VA hospitals formed the reference population from which the study subjects were selected. Three sets of criteria were met before the randomization process was implemented. The first was a set of acceptance criteria that must be met before the subject was considered eligible for participation. These included a history of stable angina pectoris for at least six months, established medical therapy program for at least three months, and electrocardiographic findings consistent with myocardial infarction or positive exercise tests. Patients who met the acceptance criteria were subjected to a set of exclusion criteria, which included acute myocardial infarction attacks in the past six months, unstable angina, or congestive heart failure. Patients who met these criteria were asked to participate in the study and sign an informed consent form. The results of angiography (visualization of the coronary arteries) were judged against a third set of criteria before final enrollment in the study. Angiographic criteria were potentially graftable condition, acceptable ventricular function, and a 50% or greater reduction in the lumen of the coronary artery.

Patients meeting these criteria were stratified on age (less than 50, and 50 and older) and whether one or two walls of the heart were involved. Each of the four stratified groups was randomized to either a medical treatment group or a surgical treatment group. The surgical group underwent saphenous vein bypass surgery. While the patency of the vessels in the surgery group were assessed at periodic intervals, all study patients were similarly followed to collect outcome data.

The first question asked was, Did the randomization work? This may be answered by carrying out a postrandomization test to compare the two groups on key variables. With the exception of serum cholesterol, which was higher in the medical than in the surgical group, factors such as history of congestive failure, hypertension, and duration of angina were quite similar in the two groups. The analysis was performed on 310 medical patients and 286 surgical patients. The two groups were also similar on the number of diseased vessels and the functioning state of the heart. The bulk of patients had triple-vessel disease and abnormal heart function.

The second question was, Did the surgical procedure work? This was answered by examining the proportion of grafted vessels that remained open and the proportion of patients with open grafts at periodic intervals. About 80% of the patients who actually underwent surgery had their coronary arteries revisualized by angiography one year on the average after surgery. It was found that 69% of all grafts were open, 54% of the patients had all of their grafts open, and 88% had at least one graft open.

The third question was, Did the surgical procedure increase survival? There was no statistically significant difference in survival between the two groups. After three years of observation, 87% of the medically treated group and 88% of the surgical bypass group were alive. Analysis of the subsets of patients who underwent surgical bypass but with double-vessel disease or triple-vessel disease and an abnormal heart function revealed no difference in survival between these two subsets and comparable subsets of patients who received medical treatment.

The results of the VA study apply only to patients with stable angina and those without left main artery obstruction. In spite of these qualifications the results of no difference between surgery and medical treatment of angina were received with mixed reactions by health professionals. It seems that "acceptance of major randomized controlled trials (RCT) by physicians depends to a large extent on whether or not they confirm or deny prior clinical judgment" (Chalmers et al. 1978). It is true that the results of the study could not be generalized to patients with chronic stable angina, left main coronary artery disease, or unstable angina. Furthermore, the results dealt strictly with survival and not the quality of life. The next set of studies contributed to knowledge in these areas.

A Subset of Patients

The improvement in the survival of patients with left main coronary artery disease as a result of saphenous vein bypass has been previously documented in a separate subgroup of the VA Cooperative Study (Takaro 1976). That subgroup of patients has been excluded from the analysis of the Veterans Administration study reviewed previously. That exclusion could have been the reason for not finding significant differences between surgery and medical treatment. Additional evidence for the better survival as a result of coronary bypass in patients with left-main coronary artery disease has been derived from a European study (European Coronary Surgery Group 1982). The Coronary Artery Surgery Study also showed that patients with left main coronary artery disease had better survival after surgical treatment (Chaitman et al. 1981). All these studies were randomized controlled trials and were consistent in providing evidence that surgery is better than medical care in the subset of patients with left main coronary artery disease.

Quality of Life

In the Coronary Artery Surgery Study, the issue of quality of life was examined (CASS 1983). Patients who underwent surgical bypass experienced less chest pain and restricted activities and required less medication. They also stayed longer on the treadmill and experienced less exercise-induced chest pain and fewer electrographic findings indicative of reduced blood supply to the heart.

Other Studies

With the exception of patients with left main coronary artery disease in whom chest pain does not respond to medical treatment, most studies have shown that surgical treatment is not better than medical intervention. Two other randomized studies have been published since the Veterans Administration study in 1977. The first was a randomized study conducted in Europe on 768 men younger than 65 years old with mild to moderate angina (European Coronary Surgery Study Group 1982). An interesting feature of that study was analyzing the two groups of patients while preserving their original group assignment. The 69 patients in the medical group who subsequently underwent surgery remained in the medical group, and the 27 patients in the surgery group who were not operated on remained in the surgery group for the purpose of the analysis.

This type of analysis offered the opportunity of testing the *policy* of deciding on surgery or medical treatment for patients. The study showed better survival for patients in the surgery group, but the bulk of the difference was shown by patients with left main coronary artery disease (survival rates of 93% compared with 62%). Medical and surgical treatments were evaluated in another controlled trial by the Coronary Artery Surgery Study Group (CASS 1983). It was concluded that surgery did not improve survival or prevent the occurrence of myocardial infarction in patients who had mild angina or who were asymptomatic after the heart attack.

Toward the Formation of Policy

The number of coronary bypass surgery operations and the cost of these operations have been challenged. Several questions have been asked: "Are the steadily increasing popularity and expense of this procedure warranted? What are the indications for CABG (Coronary Artery Bypass Grafting)? How are patients currently selected for surgery? What is the evidence that existing criteria for selection are valid?" (Braunwald 1983, p. 1181).

The results of several randomized trials on this subject should help answer some of these questions and provide rationale for policy. It is evident that the surgery is beneficial only in the subset of patients with left main coronary artery disease. It is also evident that patients who do not respond to medical treatment may benefit in terms of improved quality of life. Therefore, a policy that would entail the provision of coronary bypass surgery for such patients would be utilizing available scientific evidence. The provision of surgery for other patients would not be based on available evidence. It is believed that "this operation should and increasingly will be restricted to patients in whom intensive medical therapy has failed or in whom improved survival after surgery has been unambiguously demonstrated, rather than as a panacea for coronary artery disease" (Braunwald 1983, p. 1184).

THE COMPUTED TOMOGRAPHY (CT) SCANNER

The CT scanner is a diagnostic device that combines concepts of x-ray, television, and computers. Information obtained after the passage of an x-ray beam through the body is digitized and combined in the computer to produce images that are displayed on a television monitor. These images could be in black and white or in color. The CT scanner, developed in Great Britain in the late 1960s, is one of the many medical technologies that continue to flood the medical care scene. As with all other technologies, the application of the CT scanner in diagnosing medical problems has been the source of great enthusiasm for the medical profession but the subject of numerous discussions with regard to its impact on costs of medical care.

Interest in applying sophisticated diagnostic devices in medicine stems from several factors (U.S. Congress 1978):

- Physicians want to make an accurate diagnosis to begin with, a desire that is even more intense in the face of rising malpractice litigation.
- Although it may eventually change in the face of prospective payment, the fee-for-service system encourages the development of technologies by paying for each additional test done on a patient.

- Third party payments do not permit patients to feel directly the brunt of rising costs of medical practice (p. 6).

The efficacy and safety of CT scanners have been reviewed extensively in a 1978 publication by the Office of Technology Assessment of the U.S. Congress. It was noted that CT scanning, especially of the head, has been reliable in providing accurate diagnosis, is often used in lieu of the basic diagnostic procedures, and probably has lower risk from ionizing radiation and injected materials than the procedures it replaced. It is further noted in the report, however, that "well designed studies of efficacy of CT scanners were not conducted before widespread diffusion occurred" (p. 10).

Patterns of Use versus Efficacy Studies

In spite of a lack of studies on efficacy, the spread of CT scanners continued throughout the 1970s. Unfortunately, as is the case for most technologies, the use and popularity of a device or procedure occur before rigorous studies are done. The result is an ethical dilemma of denying a technology of presumed effi-caciousness to a group of patients (forming the control groups in a randomized trial) to generate scientific evidence for its efficacy. Furthermore, "no formal process, public or private, has existed to ensure that studies on efficacy of most technologies are conducted and that data are collected and analyzed" (U.S. Congress 1978). The impact of such information, even if available, may be minimal since "use of diagnostic technologies is not based on efficacy" and medical care standards are generally "based on accepted patterns of use rather than scientifically developed information about efficacy" (U.S. Congress 1978, p. 10).

In the *New England Journal of Medicine*, it was noted that the continued increase in physicians' enthusiasm about the procedure is matched only by continued concern about its cost (Abrams and McNeil 1978). The increased enthusiasm by physicians was largely due to their ability to make an accurate diagnosis with a noninvasive and apparently safe method. It was further noted that "the health value of a new diagnostic technology is determined by its effect on the diagnostic process, on therapy, on the course of the disease and on its outcome" (Abrams and McNeil 1978, p. 256).

The effect on the course of the disease and its outcome in terms of the occurrence of additional morbid conditions, complications, or ultimately death are important measures from an epidemiologic perspective. However, the course of disease can be changed by advances only in treatment and rehabilitation measures rather than in diagnostic accuracy alone—although making an accurate diagnosis is often a prerequisite of discovering or applying an effective treatment or rehabilitation measure. Therefore, there is no reason to expect that sophisticated diagnostic procedures including "CT of the head will statistically improve survival of patients with brain tumors in the next decade without marked changes in therapeutic efficacy" (Abrams and McNeil 1978, p. 259). However, reduced mortality and morbidity and potentially reduced costs may result from replacing invasive diagnostic methods by the noninvasive CT scanner.

Similar to CT of the head, CT of the body lacks scientific data on changing morbidity and mortality as a result of the application of the innovation. CT of the body may help in diagnosing conditions that would seem to benefit from treatment and therefore may be potentially more efficacious than CT of the head. The 1978 *New England Journal of Medicine* article concluded:

> Acceptable evidence of the efficacy of CT and in particular of its marginal contribution to diagnosis, its effect on the cost of medical care, on short-term health outcomes and on long-term health outcomes is not available. Acquisition of such data requires careful prospective studies in which the contribution of CT is clearly related to that of competing methods and the impact of additional diagnostic information is documented (Abrams and McNeil, p. 316).

Five years later an update of CT scanner technology was published (Wittenberg 1983, p. 1161). Increased sophistication in technology resulted in an increased cost of a device to about 1 million dollars. Many of the new devices scan both the head and body, collect information and reconstruct images in a much shorter time, but emit less radiation than earlier equipment. Evaluation of the CT scanner continued regarding the accuracy of the diagnosis generally and in comparison with conventional imaging tests. The impact of the CT scanner on the health state

> goes beyond the conventional quantitation of the accuracy of an examination and requires evaluation of the impact of the examination's results on clinical, diagnostic, and therapeutic decision making. The ideal study should be prospective, randomized, and comprehensive in assessing consecutive patients examined. Such an evaluation has not been carried out for CT and is unlikely to be, largely because of practical and ethical issues (Wittenberg 1983, p. 1228).

CONCLUSION

Sophistication in technology will continue, and its use will continue to spread widely in spite of escalations in medical care costs and lack of rigorous scientific evidence on the real contributions to changes in treatment modalities, improvements in physical and emotional functioning, and prolongation of survival. The emerging enthusiasm in nuclear magnetic resolution (NMR) is a good example. It is anticipated that increased interest in NMR technology may even "divert most manufacturers' efforts and resources from any large-scale advance in CT technology" (Wittenberg 1983). Policy makers are again faced with switching from one sophisticated technology to another with a momentum propelled by technological innovations rather than actual impact on improving health states of the population.

Some policy alternatives may be offered (U.S. Congress 1978):

> Alternative 1: establish a formal process to identify medical technologies that should be assessed for efficacy and safety; conduct the necessary evaluations; synthesize the results from the evaluations and from relevant clinical experience; and disseminate the resulting information to appropriate parties. Alternative 2: as part of Alternative 1, establish a formal process for making official judgments about the efficacy and safety of medical technologies. Alternative 3: authorize a federal regulatory agency, such as the Food and Drug Administration, to restrict the use of medical technologies to the conditions of use specified in the FDA-approved labelling. Alternative 4: link Medicare reimbursement to the information and judgments about the technologies' efficacy and safety that would result from Alternatives 1 and 2. Alternative 5: expand regulation of capital expenditures to cover purchases of medical equipment regardless of setting or ownership. Alternative 6: for services paid by Medicare and Medicaid, establish rates of payment that are based on efficiency. Alternative 7: fundamentally restructure the payment system to encourage providers to perform and use medical services efficiently (p. 11).

Dispassionate evaluation before widespread use of technologies is key to the resolution of this dilemma.

BIBLIOGRAPHY

Abrams HL, McNeil BJ: Medical implications of computed tomography ("CAT Scanning"). *N Engl J Med* 1978; 298(5): 255–261; 298(6): 310–318.

Banta D: Medical technology: An evolving policy issue. *Colloquium* 1982; 2(3): 1–2.

Braunwald E: Effect of coronary-artery bypass grafting on survival. Implication of the randomized coronary-artery surgery study. *N Engl J Med* 1983; 309(19): 1181–1184.

CASS Principal Investigators and Their Associates: Coronary Artery Surgery Study (CASS): A randomized trial of coronary artery bypass surgery—Quality of life in patients randomly assigned to treatment groups. *Circulation* 1983; 68: 951–960.

Chaitman BR, Fisher LD, Bourassa MG et al: Effect of coronary bypass surgery on survival patterns in subsets of patients with left main coronary artery disease. Report of the Collaborative Study in Coronary Artery Surgery (CASS). *Am J Cardiol* 1981; 48: 765–777.

Chalmers TC, Smith H, Ambroz A et al: In defense of the VA randomized control trial of coronary artery surgery. *Clinical Research* 1978; 26: 230–235.

European Coronary Surgery Study Group: Long term results of prospective randomized study of coronary artery bypass surgery in stable angina pectoris. *Lancet* 1982; 3: 1173–80.

Gaus CR: Controlling health technology. *Colloquium* 1982; 2(3): 6–7.

Harrison DC: Coronary bypass: The first 10 years. *Hospital Practice* 1981; 49–56.

Murphy ML, Hultgren HN, Detre K et al: Treatment of chronic stable angina. A preliminary report of survival data of the randomized Veterans Administration Cooperative Study. *N Engl J Med* 1977; 297: 621–627.

Russell LB: Guiding diffusion: Public policies in other countries. *Colloquium* 1982; 2(3): 3.

Showstack JA, Schroeder SA, Matsumoto MF: Changes in the use of medical technologies, 1972–77. A study of 10 inpatient diagnoses. *N Engl J Med* 1982; 306: 706–712.

Takaro T, Hultgren HN, Lipton MJ et al: The VA Cooperative Randomized Study of surgery for coronary arterial occlusive disease. II. Subgroup with significant left main lesions. *Circulation* 1976; Vol 54 No. 6 Suppl III paper II-107-III-117.

US Congress, Office of Technology Assessment: Policy implications of the computed tomography (CT) scanner. OTA-H-72 August 1978: Government Printing Office.

Wittenberg J: Computed tomography of the body. *N Engl J Med* 1983; 309(19): 1160–1165; 309(20): 1224–1229.

Chapter 11

The Health Care Professional

Several related developments concerning health care professionals emerged in the 1950s and continued through the 1960s. Physicians were unevenly distributed, especially for the delivery of medical services to rural and disadvantaged populations. There were general shortages and too much emphasis on specialization. Nurses were searching for a unique knowledge and practice base and wanted increased responsibility for patient management in addition to the traditional tasks of patient assessment. The costs of medical care were rising and were projected to increase at even faster rates. Certain groups of the population found medical care unavailable or inaccessible and many perceived it to be impersonal. In the meantime there was a strong move for increasing emphasis on primary care, general practice, and family practice. The concepts of neighborhood health centers caught the imagination of many people who advocated their rapid spread in rural and underserved areas. Health maintenance organizations (HMOs) characterized by prepayment plans and special emphasis on prevention were becoming popular.

Against this background and as one of the responses to these issues was the emergence of an expanded role in medical practice by nurse practitioners and physician assistants and associates. As their numbers increased, so did the political, economic, administrative, and licensure issues, which became the subject of controversial debates by organized medicine and nursing as well as politicians and policy makers.

One concern has been the quality of care provided by these individuals and the impact of their services on the health state of populations. Most studies on this problem were based in an office setting, and therefore their findings could not be generalized to patients with more serious acute conditions such as those found in emergency rooms or hospitals (Sox 1979). Nevertheless, these studies revealed that the quality and impact of care given by nurse practitioners were indistinguishable from that given by physicians. Many of these studies were concerned with the impact of care and were based largely on epidemiologic methods to provide the needed evidence for safety, efficacy, and effectiveness of nurse practitioners and other nonphysician personnel. An important pillar for policy making may be found by examining the results of these studies (Ibrahim 1982).

PROCESS OF MEDICAL CARE STUDIES

The estimation of the quality of medical care through the study of its processes lies within the domain of medical care research. Data on the assessment and management of a patient's condition are derived from history information, physical signs, laboratory tests, medication, and patient disposition. Process measures may be obtained from medical records or actual observations of the practice. The results are compared with explicit standards of care developed by experts under ideal conditions or a set of customary practices derived from the actual practices of clinicians. Processes of care, recorded or observed, may be judged implicitly on the basis of an evaluation of the information by a health professional or judged with reference to explicitly stated criteria. Processes-of-care studies revealed no significant differences between physicians and nurse practitioners for the care of specified conditions. Disagreements between the two were shown for a small percentage of patients whose conditions were not considered serious (Russo et al. 1975; Duncan, Smith, and Silver 1971).

In one study, clinical decision making of a pediatric nurse practitioner was tested against that of a pediatrician by reviewing the charts of 182 children with 278 conditions (Duncan, Smith, and Silver 1971). The children were seen first by the nurse practitioner and subsequently by the physician. The pediatric nurse practitioner and the pediatrician agreed on the diagnosis of conditions in 86% of the children, disagreed on insignificant conditions (such as the nurse reporting a heart murmur that the physician did not hear) in 13% of the children, and disagreed on significant conditions in the remaining 1% (or two children). The two children were diagnosed with a red sore throat by the pediatric nurse practitioner, but the pediatrician diagnosed one child as having a lower respiratory tract infection and the second as having meningitis. Inferences about these disagreements cannot be accurately made because children were not randomly assigned to the two health professionals, and furthermore the professionals apparently did not assess and manage these children independently.

In another study, every fourth child was seen by a nurse practitioner and then by a physician who did not know the nurse's evaluation. The object was to assess the triage of acute illnesses in 113 patients. No significant differences were found between the nurse practitioner and the physician (Russo et al. 1975).

The quality of the processes of medical care for selected diseases may be evaluated against the opinion of a national sample of physicians (Wagner et al. 1976, 1978). Physician responses were sought for over 100 "test situations" in reference to the diagnosis and management of an upper respiratory tract condition in a child. The physician's action may be ordering a chest x-ray or a laboratory test for the particular situation. Responses were analyzed to determine the ideal or "standard" action for a given test situation. Actual processes of care with reference to such test situations may be gathered from medical records. Comparison of the actual practice with the standard practice provides a measure of the quality of care.

Substantial discordance between what the physicians say (as expressed by responses on the questionnaire) and what they actually do (as extracted from medical records) was noted. This is exemplified by the finding that of the actions favored by the national sample of physicians for a set of test situations, only 55% actually appeared in the record (Wagner et al. 1978). The discordance varied by the nature of the action. For example, although physicians favored the recording of the absence of respiratory distress in a child with fever and cough, they did so in only 18% of such situations. The presence of a red pharynx was recorded in 86% and antibiotic treatment was recorded in 99% of cases for which physicians favored the particular action.

OUTCOME OF CARE STUDIES

Several randomized and before-after studies assessed outcome and process of health care given by practitioners other than physicians.

An Observational Study

A before-after study was conducted to evaluate the impact of a three-year nurse midwife demonstration program in Madera County, California (Levy, Wilkinson, and Marine 1971). At the county hospital two nurse midwives managed the care of about 80% of the pregnant women (after they were screened initially by a physician) and also motivated them to seek early prenatal care. Processes and outcome of care for births in the county hospital were compared with those elsewhere. About 60% of the county births belonged to the latter group.

The termination of the demonstration program after three years of operation provided an opportunity to evaluate its impact using a before-during-after design. Data from the during-program and after-program periods were compared to similar periods in the no-program patients. Prenatal clinic attendance rose during the program and declined after the program terminated (Table 11–1). First or second trimester prenatal care declined after the program terminated but remained the same in the no-program area. Six or more prenatal visits also declined after the program terminated. Prematurity declined during the program but rose after its termination, while in the no-program area a small rise was noted. While infant mortality rose after the program was terminated, with a significant rise in neonatal deaths, no substantial change was noted in the no-program area.

A cause-and-effect inference cannot be readily made from a before-after design due to the potential influence of selective and confounding biases. Nevertheless, the findings were considered persuasive by the authors of the study as to the benefits of the program, which led them to question the wisdom of discontinuing the program.

Table 11–1 Comparison of Prenatal Care and Pregnancy Outcomes between Those in the Program (County Hospital) and Those Not in the Program (Others in County)

	Program			No Program	
	Before[a]	During	After	During[b]	After[b]
Total births	345	991	768	1370	1233
Prenatal clinic attendance[c]	3.6	4.6	3.6	—	—
1st or 2nd trim. prenat. care (%)[d]	—	53.7	38.7	77.7	75.4
6 or more prenatal visits (%)[e]	—	35.3	25.1	—	—
Prematurity (%)[f]	11.0	6.6	9.8	6.0	7.4
Infant deaths (per 1,000 live births)	29.9	26.8	40.2	23.0	25.6
Fetal		29.0	22.2	27.3	17.5	17.0
Neonatal[g]		23.9	10.3	32.1	17.8	20.6
Postneonatal		6.0	16.5	8.0	5.2	5.0

Notes: [a]Duration of the before period is shorter than the during and after period. [b]During and after refer to comparable periods as in the program. [c]Ratio of annual clinic attendance to births. [d,e,f, & g]represent statistically significant differences between the during and after periods of the program.

Source: Adapted from Figure 1, Tables 1, 2, and 3, and text, B.S. Levy, F.S. Wilkinson, and W.M. Marine, "Reducing Neonatal Mortality Rate with Nurse-Midwives," *American Journal of Obstetrics and Gynecology* 109 (1): 50–58.

Randomized Trials

Certified nurse midwives who provided care to low-risk maternity patients were compared to housestaff by a randomized trial mode (Slome et al. 1976). Patients who elected to have their care provided by either housestaff or nurse midwife were excluded from the study. History of Caeserean section, diabetes, varicosities or edema, high blood pressure, and overweight were grounds for exclusion as well. The remaining patients were deemed eligible and were randomized to either the housestaff or midwives. Subsequent clinical evaluations ruled out patients with toxemias, Rh sensitivity, and other serious conditions as to receiving care from nurse midwives. Patients were followed through deliveries to determine the health state of their infants.

Prenatal care, course of delivery, and infant outcomes were found to be indistinguishable in the nurse midwife group from the housestaff group. There were only two exceptions to this finding. The first was overcompliance with appointment attendance in the nurse midwife group, and the second was a higher rate of forceps delivery by the housestaff.

The quality and impact of care by nurse practitioners were further studied in a randomized trial (Sackett et al. 1974; Spitzer et al. 1974). In this trial 1,598 families were randomized to the practice of a family physician and nurse or to a nurse practitioner. The randomization ratio was 2 to 1, respectively, for administrative (caseload) reasons. Processes of medical care were evaluated with reference to the management of 10 indicator conditions and the manner in which 13 common drugs were prescribed. A group of nonuniversity family physicians practicing in the area formulated a set of explicit criteria for what they considered adequate care.

Outcome measures included mortality, physical functioning, emotional health, and social functioning. Mortality was identified through an elaborate surveillance system specifically developed for the study. Physical functioning included measures of mobility, hearing, vision, activities of daily living, and disability. Emotional health was evaluated with regard to feelings of self-esteem, feelings toward relations with other people, and thoughts about the future. Finally, social functioning was estimated by the degree of patient's interactions and social relationships with other people and social agencies.

The differences in outcome characteristics between the practices of the nurse practitioner and the physician were not statistically significant. The processes of managing the 10 indicator conditions and prescribing the 13 common drugs were also similar in the two groups. The results of care provided by the nurse practitioner were therefore as good as those provided by the physician.

Since it was demonstrated that the practice of a health professional such as the nurse practitioner is as safe, efficacious, and effective as that of the physician, the next question may relate to cost and efficiency. An episode-based method was used to compare the efficiency of physicians with that of nurse practitioners in reference to otitis media and sore throat. The costs for episodes in which the nurse practitioner was the initial health professional seen by the patient compared favorably with those of the physicians (Salkever et al. 1982). These favorable costs were in addition to more time spent with the health professional and a larger percentage of resolved problems (Table 11–2). The findings of this study were based on the analysis of data from a group practice health maintenance organization and therefore may not be generalizable to other settings.

THE FUTURE

Indeed the economic and political considerations have played a major role in the survival of the nurse practitioner movement. In 1984, after nearly a decade, the situation was reviewed and indicated that nurse practitioners continued to be effective with no reports of harmful effects on the population served, of deterioration of health states, or of undue number of lawsuits against them. As a matter of fact, "many other innovations mediated by medical practitioners have gained widespread acceptance with less rigorous prior evaluation than was given to the use of nurse practitioners and physician assistants" (Spitzer 1984, p. 1049).

In Canada the apparent demise of the nurse practitioner movement has been attributed to the following factors (Spitzer 1984): (1) the surplus of physicians, which seems to be continuing; (2) the demand for equal pay for similar services, which is quite reasonable but negates the argument for cost containment; (3) barriers for rural and remote areas that have been operative for physicians apparently

---

Table 11–2 Process, Cost, and Outcome Measures for Otitis Media and Sore Throat Treated by Physicians or Nurse Practitioners

	Otitis Media		Sore Throat	
	MD	NP	MD	NP
Mean contact time (min.)	9.3	13.4	7.7	13.1
Percentage with lab tests	17.6	32.2	98.4	98.5
Percentage with prescriptions	84.7	91.8	59.5	58.5
Mean total costs ($)	18.2	15.0	15.6	11.8
Percentage with problem resolved	27.8	53.8	42.9	75.0

Source: Adapted from Tables 1, 4, 5, 6, D.S. Salkever, E.A. Skinner, D.M. Steinwachs et al, "Episode-Based Efficiency Comparisons for Physicians and Nurse Practitioners," Medical Care 20(2): 143–153, 1982.

continue to be operative for nurse practitioners; (4) the inability of nurse practitioners to prescribe medication independently; and (5) the unacceptance of nurse practitioners by third party payers. These factors impeded the rapid growth of the nurse practitioner movement. In Canada it seems clear that "the programs, the opportunities for practice, and concrete plans for the future are dead" (Spitzer 1984, p. 1050).

In the United States, although medical care provided by nurse practitioners is continuing, the fervor of the movement has somewhat diminished, and its future is at least uncertain. At any rate "we do not need much more research about nurse practitioners at the moment, other than surveillance. The remaining challenge is to realize the unattained but attainable benefits" (Spitzer 1984, p. 1051).

CONCLUSION

The conclusion that the performance of the nurse practitioner in specified clinical situations is safe, efficacious, effective, and efficient cannot be escaped. The clarity of evidence does not automatically mean that policy making will be easy. Health policy for the expansion and incorporation of new health professionals into the medical care system requires political and economic considerations.

BIBLIOGRAPHY

Duncan D, Smith AN, Silver HK: Comparison of the physical assessment of children by pediatric nurse practitioners and pediatricians. *Am J Pub Health* 1971; 61: 1170–1176.

Ibrahim MA: An epidemiologic perspective in health services research, in Choi T, Greenberg JN (eds): *Social Science Approaches to Health Services Research.* Ann Arbor, Mich, Health Administration Press, 1982.

Levy BS, Wilkinson FS, Marine WM: Reducing neonatal mortality rate with nurse-midwives. *Amer J Obstet Gynec* 1971; 109(1): 50–58.

Russo RM, Gururaj VJ, Bunye AS et al: Triage abilities of nurse practitioner vs pediatrician. *Am J Dis Child* 1975; 129: 673–675.

Sackett DL, Spitzer WO, Gent M et al: The Burlington randomized trial of the nurse practitioner: Health outcomes of patients. *Ann Int Med* 1974; 80: 137–142.

Salkever DS, Skinner EA, Steinwachs DM et al: Episode-based efficiency comparisons for physicians and nurse practitioners. *Med Care* 1982; 20(2): 143–153.

Slome C, Wetherbee H, Daly M et al: Effectiveness of certified nurse-midwives. A prospective evaluation study. *Am J Obstet Gynecol* 1976; 124: 177–182.

Sox HC: Quality of patient care by nurse practitioners and physician's assistants: A ten year perspective. *Ann Int Med* 1979; 91: 459–468.

Spitzer WO: The nurse practitioner revisited. Slow death of a good idea. *N Eng J Med* 1984; 310(16): 1049–1051.

Spitzer WO, Sackett DL, Sibley JC et al: The Burlington randomized trial of the nurse practitioner. *N Eng J Med* 1974; 290: 251–256.

Wagner EH, Greenberg RA, Imery PB et al: Influence of training and experience on selecting criteria to evaluate medical care. *N Eng J Med* 1976; 294: 871–876.

Wagner EH, Williams CA, Greenberg R et al: A method for selecting criteria to evaluate medical care. *Am J Public Health* 1978; 68(5): 464–470.

Part V

Health Care for Specific Conditions

Chapter 12

Coronary Heart Disease

Deaths from coronary heart and other cardiovascular diseases remain on the top of the list of causes of death in the United States and other Western countries. Indeed, cardiovascular conditions are emerging as important causes of mortality and morbidity in other countries. Interventions to curb the burdens of coronary heart disease morbidity and mortality may take place at nodal points during the clinical course of this condition. The most benefit will, of course, accrue if the condition is prevented entirely by modifying the so-called risk factors. Since not all the causes or risk factors are known, primary preventive efforts against the known risk factors cannot be expected to eradicate the condition entirely. The modification or elimination of known risk factors and causes should go a long way toward lessening the burden on society and individuals. Behavioral changes would be population based and directed toward the reduction of weight, cessation of smoking, control of high blood pressure and cholesterol, and coping with stress.

The next nodal intervention point is the out-of-hospital care. At this juncture the potential impact of mobile coronary care units or coronary care ambulances in contrast to regular emergency care should be examined. A substantial proportion of individuals will die immediately after the heart attack before coronary care ambulances can be utilized. The impact of this expensive form of care would be realized on only a small portion of the heart disease patients. The next decision after the patient survives the heart attack is whether to hospitalize or not to hospitalize and treat at home. Home care of patients with heart attacks is acceptable and practiced in the United Kingdom but is not popular in the United States.

After admission to the hospital, a number of questions may be raised with regard to the form and content of hospital care. These could involve considerable costs and psychosocial stresses on the family and patient. One issue, for example, is the use and potential benefit of certain drugs such as anticoagulants. Should the patient be admitted to a coronary care unit where care is intensive and sophisticated or admitted to regular hospital facilities for routine care? If the patient is treated in an intensive care unit, should there be early transfer to regular care? A final question relates to the length of stay in the hospital of a coronary heart disease patient and when the patient should be ambulated.

The next issue relates to care given after discharge from the hospital. Posthospital care has been almost exclusively concerned with taking medicine and having laboratory tests done at periodic intervals. Attention of the patient and physician may be focused on the psychosocial aspects resulting from a heart attack. Learning how to cope with a new situation may be as important as taking medications.

These questions have an important bearing on cost containment efforts and the diffusion of technology. When a particular procedure is adopted and assumed beneficial, its rigorous testing in a randomized controlled trial becomes an unethical and unacceptable practice since it cannot be denied to a group of patients who would serve as controls. The bias and vested interests in answering these questions may be illustrated by an anecdote that was told during the early days of a randomized controlled trial that was designed to test the benefits of home versus hospital care of coronary heart disease:

> The first report after a few months of the trial showed a slightly greater death-rate in those treated in hospital than in those treated at home. Someone reversed the figures and showed them to a CCU enthusiast who immediately declared that the trial was unethical, and must be stopped at once. When, however, he was shown the table the correct way around he could not be persuaded to declare CCUs unethical! (Cochrane 1972, p. 53)

PRIMARY PREVENTIVE MEASURES

The evidence for judging the impact of general health promotion and disease prevention measures as well as the health policy options was discussed in Chapters 8 and 9. Specific reference to elevated levels of blood pressure and blood cholesterol is found in Chapter 13.

EMERGENCY MEDICAL SERVICES

The concept of emergency medical services was apparently introduced in the late 1950s in the Soviet Union (Moiseeve 1962). The ambulances were staffed by physicians and nurses and were equipped for cardiopulmonary resuscitation. The primary aims of these units were to provide rapid response, quick transport to the nearest hospital, and administration of first aid.

In Western countries the movement to treat out-of-hospital heart patients was introduced in Belfast and New York City in the late 1960s (U.S. Department of Health and Human Services [HHS] 1981). These units were staffed by physicians and nurses and were designed to resuscitate patients with acute heart attacks. Highly trained paramedics, rather than physicians and nurses, were employed in the early 1970s to staff units in Miami, Seattle, Los Angeles, and Long Island. The increased popularity of the Regional Medical Programs in the early 1970s gave an added impetus to the use of emergency medical services. Considerable sums of money were authorized to expand emergency medical services. During all these times, no serious efforts of evaluation were conducted to judge the impact of this particular form of intervention carefully. Some individuals questioned the value of these units and thought that it should be compared with the value of educating patients not to delay in seeking care after an attack. Subsequent studies compared the effectiveness of units staffed with physicians and nurses with those staffed with paramedical personnel, rather than testing the value of providing this kind of emergency medical services to begin with.

The impact of paramedic services in which mobile intensive care units were used in contrast to regular emergency medical technician programs was studied in a suburban area around Seattle (Eisenberg, Bergner, and Hallstrom 1979). A portion of the study area of approximately 400,000 people received the emergency medical technician (EMT), and the remaining area of approximately 200,000 persons received the mobile intensive care services during a study period of 17 months between 1 April 1976 and 31 August 1977.

The lack of randomization of these areas raised a question of selection bias. The investigators compared the age distribution of heart disease deaths in the two areas and found them identical—a finding suggestive of the similarity of the two areas. The age distribution of out-of-hospital cardiac arrests due to heart disease were, however, slightly dissimilar. A greater percentage of cardiac arrests occurred in persons 80 years of age and older in the test area than in the area served by the medical technicians. In assuming that age was a predictor of survival after a cardiac arrest, it would have been expected that fewer people survived in the test area, rendering any difference found between the two areas a conservative estimate, which might not necessarily be attributable to the effect of different age distributions.

Since "information was obtained through special reports submitted by both the paramedic and EMT services" (Eisenberg, Bergner, and Hallstrom 1979, p. 41), the possibility of a reporting bias must be excluded. The out-of-hospital cardiac arrest rates due to heart disease were similar in both groups (5.6 versus 6.0), which did not support the existence of a reporting bias. An issue may be raised at this juncture as to whether the evaluation team should be different from the service team. The objectivity of an evaluation team that was not responsible for the service may be weighed against the appropriate knowledge in collecting evaluation information by the service team.

There were 301 out-of-hospital cardiac arrests due to heart disease in the EMT area compared with 186 in the test area. There were 14 survivors, or 4.7%, in the former area compared with 38, or 20.4%, in the latter area. These figures could be expressed in terms of the relative benefit (the converse of relative risk) and attributable benefit (the converse of attributable risk). The relative benefit of 4.4 (20.4% ÷ 4.7%) means that "an individual with out-of-hospital cardiac arrest was 4.4 times more likely to survive if care was given by paramedics" (Eisenberg, Bergner, and Hallstrom 1979, p. 41). An attributable benefit of about 16% (20.4% − 4.7%) means that "among 100 people with cardiac arrest in the EMT area, 16 additional individuals would have survived had paramedic services been available" (Eisenberg, Bergner, and Hallstrom, p. 41). It was concluded that these findings indicate that paramedic services (mobile coronary care units) have a "small but measurable effect on community cardiac mortality" (p. 39).

CORONARY CARE UNITS

The rapid establishment of coronary care units throughout the United States provides an excellent example in which the epidemiologic approach might have been helpful in shaping health policy. The first question is, Do coronary care units save lives? If they do, does every patient with a heart attack benefit from receiving this form of intensive care? If not, should every patient with a heart attack be admitted to a coronary care unit? If every patient does not benefit from this service and, therefore, should not be admitted to it, then who are the ones who are most likely to survive if they received intensive care? An answer to this last question will undoubtedly impact on cost of medical care, use of scarce resources, and the psychosocial and medical well-being of the patient and family.

The value of coronary care units has been addressed in the United States by analyzing death rates in hospitals before and after the introduction of coronary care units. In some instances these analyses were strengthened by comparing the results with those from control hospitals in which intensive care was not introduced at the time. Most of the studies showed that on the average the hospital death rate of coronary heart disease patients was probably reduced about 10%. Although the analysis of existing data was a commendable effort to examine the issue of the impact of coronary care units, potential biases of selection and confounding render such evaluation tenuous.

In the mid 1970s the results of a randomized controlled trial designed in England to test the impact of coronary care units were published (Mather et al. 1976). The study called for the initial recruitment of 1,895 patients from four medical centers. All were men patients younger than 70 years of age who sustained a heart attack within the previous 48 hours. About one-quarter of this group were deemed requiring mandatory hospital care. Of the remaining 1,440, 58% elected hospital care, and 11% elected home care, thereby leaving 450 patients for randomization. This group of patients, which constituted about one-quarter of the original sample, was randomized into two equal groups: one receiving home care and the other hospital care.

The reasons for excluding patients from the clinical trial were mandatory hospital care, opting strongly for either home or hospital care, individuals with inadequate care at home, or patients who were considered by their physicians to have medical conditions that might have been associated with their heart attacks.

The two randomized groups were found comparable on age, history of angina pectoris, history of infarction, hypertension, and diabetes. In addition, the two groups were comparable on the length of time between onset of the condition and receipt of medical care. The two groups were therefore similar in most respects with the exception of the mode of treatment: home versus hospital. The difference in death rates between the hospital-treated and the home-treated patients was not statistically significant (Table 12–1). Of special interest was the fact that most patients who were 60 years of age and older without low levels of blood pressure (hypotension) had indeed a lower death rate if treated at home than similar patients who were treated at the hospital.

Table 12–1 Death Rates in Heart Attack Patients Randomly Treated at Home or Hospital

	Death Rates Percentages	
	Random Home (n = 226)	*Random Hospital* (n = 224)
< 1 week	4	7
< 1 year		
Total	23	30
<60	17	18
60 +	23	35
Hypotension		
Present	56	43
Absent	16	25
Absent in 60 +	16	31

Source: Adapted from H.G. Mather, D.C. Morgan, N.G. Pearson et al., "Myocardial Infarction: A Comparison between Home and Hospital Care for Patients," *British Medical Journal* 1976 (1): 925–929.

In this study only one-quarter of the eligible patients were randomized, and therefore generalizability of the findings of no difference between home and hospital care was limited to only that group of patients. Nevertheless, the information should provide a good scientific basis for the proper use of resources for at least one-quarter of eligible patients—not an insignificant segment. In another study three-quarters of eligible patients with confirmed heart attacks in Nottingham were randomized to home or hospital care (Hill, Hampton, and Mitchell 1978). The six-week death rate in the two groups did not differ significantly, indicating that hospital care did not offer specific advantages for survival when compared with care given at home.

Beneficiaries and Circumstances

Inspired by such findings, but faced with the impractical option of treating heart attack patients at home, American physicians began to ask a different question: What patients benefit most from intensive care, and under what circumstances, and what patients could be transferred early to routine care? The development of specific predictors of mortality (during hospital stay and beyond) and complications is necessary to answer such questions.

Analysis of existing data revealed that patients could be classified into various degrees of risk according to demographic and diagnostic criteria. A small proportion of the patients in the "low-risk" group would require intensive care (Fuchs and Scheidt 1981). Furthermore, the relative absence of complications and death in the low-risk patients compared with intermediate- or high-risk patients may provide the basis for early transfer of such patients to routine care, thereby reducing by 55% the total number of days that such patients would have to spend in an intensive care unit (Mulley et al. 1980). This inference was based on analysis of existing data on 360 patients. It requires further testing by a randomized controlled trial to provide a firm evidence for making policy.

The relentless quest for containing costs but providing quality care continues. A substantial portion, probably 50%, of the patients presenting in an emergency room with symptoms indicative of potential heart attack will eventually have a diagnosis of no heart attack. If this group of patients is identified and treated in other than intensive care facilities, a considerable amount of resources could be saved. Assuming that this segment could be identified, various alternative strategies of management could be tested, using the modeling approach discussed in Chapter 5. The clinical and economic consequences of alternative management strategies were examined (Fineberg, Scadden, and Goldman 1984). The four strategies included admitting patients to an intensive coronary care unit, to an intermediate care unit, to routine hospital care, or to care provided as an outpatient. The calculations in the model applied to patients received in emergency rooms with acute chest pain who are expected to develop definite myocardial infarction with a probability of about 5%. Estimates of complications, early mortality, long-term survival, and economic costs were calculated from available studies.

The results indicated that coronary care units would save 145 lives in a year but at an extra cost of $297 million as compared with an intermediate level of care. Although extra savings could be realized by providing routine medical care or outpatient care, this would occur at the expense of losing an unacceptable number of lives. This modeling approach suggested that many patients who have a low probability of developing definitive heart attack may be appropriately placed at lesser cost and without unduly increased risk of mortality in an intermediate care facility.

Determining the probability of developing an acute heart attack in patients presenting themselves to an emergency room would aid the physician in deciding whether to admit the patient to a coronary care unit. Such an instrument was developed from data on about 2,800 patients in six New England hospitals, allowing for a probability score to be computed with a programmable calculator (Pozen et al. 1984). The validity of using this instrument for the accuracy of the diagnosis and subsequent admission to coronary care unit was determined in a prospective trial on 2,320 patients (Pozen et al. 1984). The probability score for each patient was made available to the physician during the experimental period of study, but the physician was free to make a decision to admit on the basis of that score or on personal judgment without reference to the score. The probability of developing an acute heart attack was calculated on all patients during the control period of the study but was not made available to the physician.

In comparing the control with the experimental period, it was found that the diagnostic accuracy increased from 79.6% to 83.4%, the false positive diagnosis rate decreased from 41% to 32.8%, and the false negative diagnosis rate increased from 2.5% to 3.3%. In addition, the final diagnosis of negative heart disease decreased from 24% to 17%. This represented a decrease of 30% of those who eventually would have been found not to have the disease. It was estimated that the use of such an instrument could reduce the number of admissions to coronary care units in the entire country by about 250,000 per year (Pozen et al. 1984).

These studies and predictive models and instruments that were developed to deal with the issue of admission to coronary care units are of utmost importance. They clearly point the way for using scientific information in decision making that would contain costs and allocate resources properly and without endangering the health state of the population.

EARLY HOSPITAL MOBILIZATION AND DISCHARGE

Efforts to get patients out of hospital beds sooner and discharge them earlier than what used to be usual practice are considered good medicine, and also good measures to reduce costs of hospital care. Patients with coronary heart disease once were hospitalized for at least five or six weeks with very little activity during hospitalization, followed by a period of cautious return to normal activities. In order to test the possible benefit of early mobilization, male patients with acute myocardial infarction were allocated on consecutive days to one or another of two groups: regular mobilization of five weeks' duration or early mobilization of three weeks' duration (Groden 1971). The two groups were similar on mean age and distribution of the Peel Index, a prognostic measure of mortality among coronary heart disease patients. The latter index was relevant for comparing the two groups since the hypothesis to be tested was concerned with prognosis.

In some studies with similar purposes, comparisons are often made on risk rather than prognostic factors. Although it is desirable to have the two groups comparable on risk factors as well, the consequences of coronary heart disease represent the end results in this case, and therefore prognostic factors, such as those combined in the Peel Index, would be the more relevant to use.

Patients in the two groups were managed in a similar fashion except for mobilization management during their hospital stay. During the first week while patients in the regular mobilization group were put to total bed rest and fed and washed by a nurse for three days, patients in the early mobilization group assumed a comfortable position in bed and fed or washed themselves. In the second week patients in the regular mobilization group engaged in practices similar to the first week of the early mobilization group while that group continued the pattern started in the first week. In the third week patients in the regular mobilization group assumed a comfortable position in bed, while those in the early mobilization group began to move around and were given toilet privilege. On the twenty-second day the early mobilization group patients were allowed to go home, while the other group continued hospitalization until discharge on the thirty-sixth day. The documentation of services provided in this study is noteworthy.

No significant differences were noted between these two groups with regard to any of the following outcome variables: mortality, further pain, disturbed rhythm, psychosocial disturbances, or return to work (Table 12–2). The conclusion that early mobilization had no adverse effects on the health of patients with myocardial infarction provided a sound basis for reducing the length of hospital stay. Cost containment efforts should be easily realized by reducing hospital stay an average of two weeks.

Seven years after these results were published, the notion of discharging patients one week after acute myocardial infarction was tested (McNeer et al. 1978). The study population consisted of 67 consecutive patients who had no serious complications by the fifth hospital day. These patients were free of ventricular tachycardia or fibrillation, second- or third-degree heart block, pulmonary edema, or persistent hypotension. In addition, these were patients who had a conducive home environment permitting regular checkups and visits by a specially trained

Table 12–2 Outcomes in Regular and Early Mobilization Groups

	Regular Mobilization (N = 55)	Early Mobilization (N = 50)
Complications (percentage in each group)		
Hospital deaths	22	18
Episodes of pain after original M.I.	27	32
Arrhythmia	33	38
Psychological disturbances in hospital	9	10
Psychological disturbances in hospital or after		
return home	26	28
Return to work (percentage of those classified as fit for work)		
Working at 3 months	39	54
Working at 4 months*	52	81
Working at 5 months*	52	81
Working at 6 months	71	88

Note: *$P < .05$

Source: Adapted from Tables 1 and 2, B.M. Groden, "The Management of Myocardial Infarction. A Controlled Study of the Effects of Early Mobilization," *Cardiac Rehabilitation* 1(4): 13–16.

nurse practitioner. Half of these patients were discharged at one week, and the other half discharged between one and three weeks. The two groups were comparable on age, race, sex, history of angina, and other characteristics.

No significant differences were noted in the two groups with reference to death, recurrent infarction, chest pain, congestive heart failure, or return to work (McNeer et al. 1978). A net saving per patient of about $2,000 in 1977 prices in addition to the comfort of being home in a familiar environment with family and friends was realized.

Early mobilization and discharge were also tested on 189 patients with uncomplicated myocardial infarction (Hayes, Morris, and Hampton 1974). These patients were randomized into an early or late mobilization and discharge group. Patients in the first groups were mobilized immediately and discharged after nine days of hospitalization, while the second group was mobilized on the ninth day and discharged after two weeks. The two groups were similar on baseline characteristics. No significant differences were noted between the two groups with regard to recurrent chest pain, myocardial infarction, heart failure, or disturbed rhythm.

POSTHOSPITAL CARE

After hospital discharge, patients who had suffered acute myocardial infarction generally receive regular medical care, which is mostly concerned with taking and adhering to prescribed drugs. The well-recognized psychosocial impact of the condition on the patient and family led to studies in which measures of coping with the new circumstances created by the patient's condition are tested. Emotional problems often complicate the patient's life and create conflicts among family members and interfere with return to meaningful work. Denial of such problems is often characteristic of patients who have had heart attacks.

One form of affordable intervention might be in the provision of the so-called group psychotherapy for heart attack patients. The evidence from the various studies published so far is persuasive but not yet conclusive. The potential benefits of group psychotherapy have been studied by different investigators and have shown relatively consistent results (Ibrahim 1976). Although the number of patients in each psychotherapy group, the length of each session, the number of sessions, the mix of patients, and the background of group leaders differed, the results indicate that this form of intervention is acceptable, easy to adhere to, and helpful to patients in adapting and coping with the new circumstances created by their condition. Frequency of chest pains, frequency and length of hospitalization, depression states, and anxieties improved with this form of intervention rather than without it.

This seemingly useful approach to management of patients with heart attacks, which evidently requires further research, is worthy of consideration in the total treatment plan for this condition. The incorporation of this form of therapy may have a bearing on the quality of life of patients and their families and on containment of medical care costs as a result of reduced rehospitalizations and length of stay as well as return to gainful employment.

CONCLUSION

The spectrum of health and medical care for coronary heart disease is exemplified by tracing the clinical course of this condition, beginning with primary prevention and ending with posthospital care. Primary prevention directed toward the modification of known risk factors in the population would reduce the incidence of coronary heart disease and potentially reduce its considerable burdens on society. Programs established for this purpose would represent efficient use of resources. The major limitations in this regard are the lack of adequate knowledge on all the risk factors and the value of intervention measures on reducing the risk of acquiring the disease.

The second phase in the provision of appropriate care for coronary heart disease patients is the reduction of out-of-hospital deaths. Once the heart attack occurs, up to one-half of those who suffer the attack cannot be helped and die suddenly. Those who do not die suddenly are candidates for rapid transport to an emergency facility. The coronary care mobile unit would seem to save about 15% of this group.

The third phase in the clinical course of the disease is the admission to a coronary care unit. About one-half of those who avail themselves for admission to a coronary care unit complaining of chest pain would be ruled out eventually as not having coronary heart disease. Development of criteria for screening out this group would save resources.

The fourth point on the clinical course of coronary heart disease is early ambulation of the patient, reduced length of hospital stay, and early transfer from a coronary care unit or early discharge from the hospital altogether. These should have implications on cost as well as family and patient quality of life. The final phase is posthospital care, which could prudently include activities directed toward coping with the psychosocial circumstances resulting from the attack.

Efforts to reduce the burden of coronary heart disease on the population stretch from changing life styles, providing various forms of therapy, and introducing new and expensive technologies such as coronary care mobile units and hospital coronary care units. The formulation of health policy to deal with this complex spectrum may be aided by the study of the scientific evidence available. Some, however, believe that "cost containment efforts will fail if they continue to ignore the structural relationships between health care costs and private profit in capitalist society . . . cost-effective methodology obscures the profit motive as a basic source of high costs and ineffective practices" (Waitzkin 1979, p. 1260). Others would argue that "it is not a desire for profit that is linked to rising costs, but the lack of competition among providers, and the absence of a link between profits and the efficient (lowest unit cost) use of resources and technologies whose effectiveness has been proven" (Bloom 1979, p. 1271). The truth perhaps lies between these two positions.

BIBLIOGRAPHY

Bloom BS: Stretching ideology to the utmost: Marxism and medical technology. *Amer J Pub Health* 1979; 69(12): 1269–1271.

Cochrane AL: *Effectiveness and Efficiency—Random Reflections on Health Services*. London, Nuffield Provisional Hospitals Trust, 1972, p 53.

Eisenberg M, Bergner L, Hallstrom A: Paramedic programs and out-of-hospital cardiac arrests: II. Impact on community mortality. *Am J Public Health* 1979; 69: 39–42.

Fineberg HV, Scadden D, Goldman L: Care of patients with a low probability of acute myocardial infarction. Cost effectiveness of alternatives to coronary-care-unit admission. *N Engl J Med* 1984; 310: 1301–1307.

Fuchs R, Scheidt S: Improved criteria for admission to cardiac care units. *JAMA* 1981; 246: 2037–2041.

Groden BM: The management of myocardial infarction. A controlled study of the effects of early mobilization. *Cardiac Rehab* 1971; 1(4): 13–16.

Hayes MJ, Morris GK, Hampton JR: Comparison of mobilization after two and nine days in uncomplicated myocardial infarction. *Brit Med J* 1974; 3: 10–13.

Hill JD, Hampton JR, Mitchell JRA: A randomized trial of home-versus-hospital management for patients with suspected myocardial infarction. *Lancet* 1978; 1: 837–841.

Ibrahim MA: The impact of intervention upon psychosocial functions of postmyocardial infarction patients. *J S Carol Med Asso* 1976; 72 (suppl): 23–26.

Mather HG, Morgan DC, Pearson NG et al: Myocardial infarction: A comparison between home and hospital care for patients. *Brit Med J* 1976; 1: 925–929.

McNeer JF, Wagner GS, Ginsburg PB et al: Hospital discharge one week after acute myocardial infarction. *N Engl J Med* 1978; 298: 229–232.

Moiseeve SG: Experience in the administration of first aid to patients with myocardial infarction in Moscow. *Soviet Med*, June 1962; 26: 30–35.

Mulley AG, Thibault GE, Hughes RA et al: The course of patients with suspected myocardial infarction. The identification of low-risk patients for early transfer from intensive care. *N Engl J Med* 1980; 302: 943–948.

National Center for Health Services Research: Evaluation of Paramedic Services for Cardiac Arrest, US Dept of Health and Human Services publication No. (PHS) 82–3310, December 1981.

Pozen MW, D'Agostino RB, Selker HP et al: A predictive instrument to improve coronary-care-unit admission practices in acute ischemic heart disease. A prospective multicenter clinical trial. *N Eng J Med* 1984; 310: 1273–1278.

Waitzkin H: A Marxian interpretation of the growth and development of coronary care technology. *Amer J Pub Health* 1979; 69(12): 1260–1268.

Chapter 13

High Blood Pressure and Blood Cholesterol

Research efforts to combat cardiovascular diseases range from those at the basic level on the human cell and body fluids to those at the population level or epidemiologic investigations of risk factors. Epidemiologic methods and principles are best exemplified by their application to the field of cardiovascular disease. Descriptive studies of mortality, continuing since the turn of the century, were instrumental in identifying geographic areas at high risk as well as segments of the population most prone to dying from coronary heart disease. Several case-control studies were carried out in the 1940s, 1950s, and 1960s to identify specific risk factors.

It was not until the well-known prospective Framingham Heart Study, which began in the late 1940s and early 1950s, that the scientific community and the public were provided with a list of the so-called coronary heart disease risk factors. These included elevated levels of blood pressure and blood cholesterol, cigarette smoking, overweight, and lack of physical activities. The identification of these risk factors led to a number of clinical and community randomized trials that were conducted in the 1970s in order to estimate the consequences of changing the risk factors. While many of these intervention trials were ongoing, a number of intervention programs were introduced, occasionally by the same government agencies that are conducting the intervention trials. The three distinct stages of development in the cardiovascular disease field—the identification of risk factors, the design and conduct of intervention trials, and the implementation of control programs—offered the scientific community, the public, and the policy makers exciting opportunities for debates on several policy issues.

HIGH BLOOD PRESSURE

The magnitude of high blood pressure in the American population varies according to the level of blood pressure chosen. At a diastolic blood pressure level of 90 mm Hg or higher, about 60 million Americans are affected. The condition is prevalent among men and women, blacks and whites, and young and old. It is, however, more prevalent (and perhaps more serious) among the black than the white population of the United States.

Although epidemiologic studies revealed the association between increased levels of blood pressure and increased mortality "it does not necessarily follow from these observations that lowering arterial pressure will prolong life, but it strongly encourages the research worker to use RCTs to test the hypothesis" (Cochrane 1972, p. 49). Randomized controlled trials (RCTs) were forthcoming. A clinical randomized controlled trial in the Veterans Administration hospital patients was designed to test the efficacy of treating high blood pressure with medication (Veterans Administration Cooperative Study Group 1970). This study showed that antihypertensive medication conferred a good measure of protection against dying among a selected group of male veterans who complied with medication and clinic attendance. The results of this carefully conducted clinical trial in a hospital setting led the way to community-based studies.

Drug Treatment of Mild Hypertension

The Hypertension Detection and Follow-up Program (HDFP) is one of the most publicized community-based controlled trials (Hypertension Detection and Follow-up Program Cooperative Group 1979). The study was designed to test the impact of step-care programs on mortality in contrast with regular community care. The population consisted of about 11,000 individuals with diastolic blood pressure of 90 mm Hg or higher who were recruited from 14 centers in the United States. The two groups (step-care and regular care) were different not only in the treatment regimen against high blood pressure but also in the availability and cost of medical care. The step-care group received care at no cost while the other group received care at usual costs. Random assignments into the two groups were made within blood pressure level subgroups of 90–104, 105–114, and 115+ mm Hg. The study showed the benefit of the step-care in that the five-year mortality from all causes was reduced 17% in that group compared with the regular care group.

The Australian study involved fewer individuals (about 3,500) than the HDFP, with individual diastolic blood pressure ranging from 95 to 109 mm Hg (Management Committee of the Australian Hypertension Trial 1980). The two groups received identical care (unlike the HDFP) except for the antihypertensive medication. The results indicated that drug treatment of hypertension (including mild hypertension beginning at 95 diastolic) was associated with reduction of mortality and morbidity from cardiovascular diseases. In other words this study agreed with the HDFP, except that it did not include patients with diastolic blood pressure levels between 90 and 94 mm Hg.

The evidence in favor of treating mild hypertensives was not clearly shown in other trials. In spite of a reduction in blood pressure levels, the Oslo study showed no difference in morbidity or mortality between patients treated by active drugs compared to a control group (Helgeland 1980). The Oslo study confirmed other studies that showed no significant difference between active treatment by drugs of mild hypertensives and treatment by a placebo (Veterans Administration Cooperative Study Group on Antihypertensive Agents 1970; Smith 1977). The significant findings shown in the HDFP in the treatment of mild hypertensives, which was confirmed by the Australian study (except for individuals with diastolic blood pressure between 90 and 95), and the negative findings of the other studies created a dilemma for practicing physicians who were seeking policy guidelines on the care of their patients.

It would seem that "the evidence supporting the value of treating borderline and mild hypertension with antihypertensive drugs, therefore, is not as clearly established as many believe" (Freis 1982). The question of the impact of quality medical care generally compared with specific drug treatment for hypertension continues to be raised with regard to the results of the HDFP. Other studies that were specifically designed to test the efficacy of drug treatment showed equivocal results. It is well known that the risk of heart attacks increases with the presence of other risk factors. It may be assumed therefore that antihypertensive treatment would be "most beneficial in patients with multiple risk factors" (Freis 1982). In view of these questions, a compromise position may be adopted in that "patients with diastolic pressures of 90–99 mm Hg (average of at least three visits) are treated or not, according to the number of risk factors present. Patients with few other risk factors are given reducing or low-sodium diets but not drugs" (Freis 1982).

Treatment of mild hypertension by nonpharmacologic means has been gaining momentum. Nonpharmacologic means include reduction of body weight, sodium intake, alcohol, fats, and tobacco consumption; engagement in physical activity; and application of some form of behavioral modification. The most recent policy on the treatment of mild hypertension makes a distinction between those under and those above the level of 95 mm Hg:

> The benefits of drug therapy seem to outweigh any known risks from such therapy for those with a diastolic BP persistently elevated above 95 mm Hg and for those with lesser elevation who are at high risk. . . . For those with diastolic BPs in the 90- to 94–mm Hg range who are otherwise at low risk, nonpharmacologic therapy should be pursued aggressively while BPs are carefully monitored. (The Joint National

Committee on Detection, Evaluation, and Treatment of High Blood
Pressure 1984, p. 1049)

The classifications and definitions of hypertension were reexamined by the 1984
joint national committee in an effort to establish categories that are not only widely
accepted but indicative of an explicit follow-up and management plans. Reaffir-
mation was given to the importance of diastolic blood pressure level in labeling
mild (90–104), moderate (105–114), and severe (115+) hypertension. When
diastolic blood pressure level is less than 90 mm Hg, systolic blood pressure level
bears significance in labeling individuals as borderline isolated systolic hypertensives (140–159) or isolated systolic hypertensives (160+).

Of specific importance is the agreement that diastolic hypertension must not be
extended to levels of diastolic blood pressure below 90 mm Hg; individuals with
levels between 85 and 89 should be designated as high normals, subjected to
surveillance, and advised about nonpharmacologic measures. This stand coupled
with the policy as quoted with reference to patients with mild hypertension
(diastolic blood pressures of 90 to 94 and 95 to 104) should discourage the
widespread and indiscriminate use of antihypertensive drugs.

Other Issues in Hypertension

Two other policy issues with regard to the detection and treatment of high blood
pressure are worthy of note. Should door-to-door screening programs to identify
those with high blood pressure be continued? Such programs were fashionable
years ago even though their effectiveness in identifying new patients with elevated
levels of high blood pressure was questioned. With the increased accessibility to
medical care, the increased awareness about high blood pressure among professionals as well as the public, and the fact that most people will be seen by a
physician during the course of two to three years, it is generally agreed that blood
pressure detection and treatment should be carried out in primary care settings.
Funds spent on door-to-door screening for high blood pressure or for measuring
blood pressures in settings other than health care (such as shopping malls) should
be discouraged.

Another important question is, When does the evidence become sufficient to
recommend implementation of intervention programs? The National Heart, Lung,
and Blood Institute launched two major efforts in 1971. The first was the creation
of the National High Blood Pressure Education Program, which was designed to
"inform the public and health care professionals about the facts and opportunities
on hand about high blood pressure so as to stimulate more awareness and
aggressive treatment of the disease" (Levy 1979, p. 2). The second was the establishment of the Multicenter Hypertension Detection and Follow-up Program, which

was designed to "gain additional facts and to resolve unsettled issues regarding the treatment of high blood pressure" (Levy 1979).

These may seem to be two contradictory statements. One advocates aggressive treatment of high blood pressure, and the other seeks more knowledge about the impact of treatment of high blood pressure. The statements seem to represent a compromise stand by the National Heart, Lung, and Blood Institute in the face of the need to do something with the information available and the need to collect better evidence for the formulation of a sound policy. Some would say that the National Heart, Lung, and Blood Institute should have delayed the implementation of intervention programs until the results of its multicenter controlled community trials became available. Others would say that the controlled trials would produce evidence already established by less rigorous and less expensive studies. Perhaps the stand by the National Heart, Lung, and Blood Institute in 1972 represented a reasonable policy on the matter.

HIGH BLOOD CHOLESTEROL

Diets high in saturated fats and cholesterol are associated with increased morbidity rates of coronary heart disease as well as an increased risk of dying from it. The association was particularly evident in ecologic studies in which the degree of saturated fat consumption per capita of several countries was found to be directly correlated with the frequency of heart attacks in those countries (Keys 1970). These ecologic studies revealed that as the percentage of saturated fat in the diets increased, so did the frequency of heart attacks. Scientific evidence obtained from ecologic studies is considered suggestive of causal relationships, as discussed in Chapter 4. It cannot be construed to provide sufficient grounds for firm causal inferences. For various reasons, including the absence of meaningful differences in dietary habits of a population, relationships between saturated fat percentages in diets and coronary heart disease have not been shown within a particular country.

The causal role of high levels of blood cholesterol in the development of and death from coronary heart disease has been persuasively established in prospective epidemiologic studies such as the Framingham Heart Study. Several studies have confirmed such a relationship and there is now general agreement among scientists that increased levels of blood cholesterol are "causally" related to heart attacks. More sophisticated studies have shown that a special component of cholesterol known as low-density lipoprotein (LDL) is the fraction that is related to heart attacks and is indeed related to dietary fat intake. Another fraction of the cholesterol known as high-density lipoprotein (HDL) is shown to be inversely related to coronary heart disease and therefore may be considered a "protective" factor. It has been shown that HDL is also associated with physical activity, smoking cessation, and moderate alcohol consumption.

Although the proposition that high saturated fats and cholesterol in the diet, as well as high blood cholesterol, are associated with an increased risk of coronary heart disease, the question that needs to be answered is, Would reducing saturated fats and cholesterol in the diet or reducing blood cholesterol with diets or cholesterol-lowering drugs be associated with a reduction in the risk of heart attacks? For some time there has been no good answer to this question. Fragmentary evidence has been available from studies on individuals who changed their homeland, such as the Japanese, but maintained dietary habits that are low in saturated fats, and on vegetarians such as the Seventh-Day Adventists. These observations provided good clues as to the impact of diets low in saturated fats but did not provide sufficient evidence for a firm stand on this issue or recommendations for dietary changes.

Against this background of scientific findings, an interplay flourished among nutritionists, the government and its scientists, and the powerful dairy, egg, and meat lobbies (Hausman 1981). The long-standing emphasis by nutritionists on the nutrient value of foods and their advocacy for the so-called basic four food groups—dairy, meat, fruit and vegetables, and breads and cereals—seemed to interfere with their accepting the widely publicized potential harmful effects of saturated fats and cholesterol on people;

> The heart researchers' conclusions couldn't have been a bigger affront to the basic commitment of nutritionists: the Basic Four. It was a challenge not just to commonly accepted notions about the most nutritious foods, but also to the most fundamental assumption in nutrition: *that nutrition is the study of the beneficial elements in food.* (Hausman 1981, p 32)

Arguments to belittle the relationship were advanced in much the same vein as the argument to belittle the relationship between smoking and lung cancer. For example,

> the diets lower in saturated fat and cholesterol prevent heart disease, but cause malnutrition instead . . . lack of exercise is a more important cause of heart disease than diet . . . blood cholesterol levels can only be lowered 10 to 15 percent—a trivial amount . . . there is no proof that lowering blood cholesterol levels will prevent heart disease. (Hausman 1981, pp. 72, 79, 81, 87)

There is some truth to some of these arguments, especially the last assertion, until the results of the Lipid Research Clinics Program were published, which are discussed later.

Government agencies including the National Institutes of Health were not immune to resisting change. The "Federal Turtle," as has been characterized by some (Hausman 1981), was exemplified in 1965 by the Food and Drug Administration proposing labels to indicate the type of fat in foods, subsequently tabling that proposal, and finally adopting it in 1973; or the National Heart, Lung, and Blood Institute rejection of a report developed by a task force in 1971 that advised Americans to lower their intake of cholesterol and dietary saturated fats (Hausman 1981).

The various lobbies played their roles as well. The meat lobby, for example, spoke vigorously against any scientific information incriminating meat as a factor in coronary heart disease. They widely advertised reports by scientists, especially nutritionists, that were against dietary changes. They lobbied vigorously against any change in dietary habits and "continued to assure their constituents that the evidence against saturated fat was slim" (Hausman 1981, p. 187).

Likewise, the dairy lobby used its considerable political influence to convince its constituents that fat in milk is not detrimental to health and continued to wage war against the American Heart Association position. One of the tactics "to diffuse concern about milk fat is acknowledging only its cholesterol but not its saturated fat. This strategy ". . . can fool people who associate only cholesterol in food with cholesterol in the blood, unaware that saturated fat is the prime influence on blood cholesterol levels" (Hausman 1981, p. 208). The egg producers and their lobbyists acted in a similar fashion to other groups. They attempted to influence government agencies and Congress in ways to make them reject the relationship between cholesterol in eggs and heart disease and to oppose the American Heart Association's stand on these matters.

Then came the evidence of a randomized trial that was specifically designed to answer the question of whether reducing blood cholesterol by diet or cholesterol-lowering drugs would result in reduction of coronary heart disease.

A Randomized Trial

Testing the efficacy of a cholesterol-lowering diet is impractical because such a diet would reduce cholesterol by a small amount and therefore require a large number of people to show an effect. In addition, it would be difficult to maintain unawareness on the part of the study subjects as to the nature of the experiment, and therefore a bias may be introduced in the study. A cholesterol-lowering drug that is safe and nonabsorbent, that works on the intestine mimicking the action of diet, would be ideal especially if given to individuals with high levels of blood cholesterol, therefore allowing the execution of an experiment on a relatively small sample size.

The Lipid Research Clinics Program conducted such an experiment in 12 centers in North America (Lipid Research Clinics Program I and II 1984). In this trial about 3,800 men aged 35 to 59 with blood cholesterol levels above 265 milligrams but with no evidence of coronary heart disease were chosen for the experiment. These men were recruited from more than 400,000 men who were initially screened, but a substantial number of them were excluded because of such characteristics as high blood pressure, symptoms of coronary heart disease, or other major illnesses. Those considered for the study (18,000) underwent a period of prerandomization when their willingness to consume diets low in cholesterol, their appointment-keeping behavior, and their attitude toward participation and long-term commitment to the study were assessed. After careful review, 3,806 men were selected to participate in the study and were randomized into a cholesterol-lowering drug group and a placebo group. Both groups continued to receive dietary instructions designed to encourage them to consume diets low in cholesterol content. The two groups were similar on key characteristics and were followed for an average of 10 years.

Coronary heart disease events (coronary heart disease deaths and nonfatal heart attacks) occurred with a frequency of 187 in the placebo group compared with 155 in the treatment group resulting in a reduction of 19% (Table 13–1). If only coronary heart disease deaths were considered, the reduction was about 24%. There was a reduction of only 7% in the all-deaths category, but deaths from accidents and violence occurred with a larger frequency in the cholesterol-lowering drug group than in the placebo group (11 versus 4 deaths). Underlying coronary heart disease, events were ruled out in all the deaths due to accidents and violence, and it was concluded after careful examination that the difference between the two groups was due to a chance occurrence. Other manifestations of coronary heart disease such as positive exercise tests, angina pectoris, or coronary bypass surgery were reduced in the cholesterol-lowering drug group 20 to 25% in comparison with the placebo group.

As described in Chapter 1, evaluation research requires the identification of the process as well as the change that would be expected to result from it, and the relationship of the change to the outcome. In this trial it was shown that the two groups generally followed their diets (the process) as demonstrated by the similarities between them in total calories, dietary cholesterol, and the polyunsaturated/saturated fats ratio (Table 13–2). Total blood cholesterol and LDL cholesterol were reduced (the changes) about 20 milligrams on the average in the cholesterol-lowering drug group compared with the placebo group. The associated outcome, as described, was a reduction in coronary heart disease mortality and morbidity.

Table 13–1 Lowering of Cholesterol and the Occurrence of Coronary Heart Disease after Seven Years of Follow-up

	Placebo Group (n = 1,900)	*Cholesterol-lowering Drug Group (n = 1,906)*	*% Reduction in risk[a]*
All CHD events	187	155	19
CHD deaths	38	30	24
Accidents & violence	4	11	—
All deaths	71	68	7
Positive exercise test	345	260	25
Angina pectoris	287	235	20
Coronary bypass	112	93	21

[a]Percentage of reduction is adjusted for follow-up time and stratification.

Source: Adapted from Tables 3 and 4, Lipid Research Clinics Program, "The Lipid Research Clinics Coronary Primary Prevention Trial Results," *JAMA* 1984 (251): 365–374. Copyright 1984 by the American Medical Association.

Table 13–2 Dietary Intake, Changes in Cholesterol, and Dose-Response Relationship at End of Study

	Placebo Group	*Cholesterol-lowering Drug Group*
Total calories	2,060	2,086
Cholesterol, mg	284	288
P/S ratio	0.67	0.66
Total cholesterol	277.3	257.1
LDL cholesterol	197.6	174.9
0–1 packet/day		
% reduction, cholesterol	−3.2	−3.9
% reduction, LDL	−4.8	−6.6
> 5 packet/day		
% reduction, cholesterol	−5.4	−19.0
% reduction, LDL	−8.4	−28.3

Source: Adapted from Tables 1 and 2, p. 354, and Table 1, p. 369, Lipid Research Clinics Program, "The Lipid Research Clinics Coronary Primary Prevention Trial Results," *JAMA* 1984 (251): 351–364 and II 365–374. Copyright 1984 by the American Medical Association.

Furthermore, the magnitude of reduction in cholesterol and LDL cholesterol was related to the number of packets consumed per day. A dose-response relationship such as this further strengthens a causal relationship, as outlined in Chapter 4. Although there was some relationship in the placebo group, a considerable gradient was shown in the treatment group. For example, the percentage of reduction in cholesterol increased from -3.9% in those individuals consuming up to one packet per day to -19% in those consuming five packets or more (Table 13-2).

This trial showed that cholesterol can be lowered in individuals by dietary means as well as cholesterol-lowering drugs, that individuals do adhere to such a regimen, that reduction in cholesterol and adherence to the drug or dietary regimen are associated with reduction in coronary heart disease, and that the degree of adherence is associated with the degree of reduction in the disease. The randomized nature of this study, the clear difference between the two groups, and the demonstration of a dose-response relationship indicate that the results should provide firm evidence for the association between reduction of cholesterol and reduced frequency of coronary heart disease. The applicability of these findings to women, younger men, and individuals with lower levels of cholesterol should be further examined as this study does not provide direct evidence in this regard.

Evidence and Policy

In spite of this firm evidence, the dairy representative on a Sunday newsmaker show on cable television on May 7, 1984, claimed that dairy products are the "best foods for longevity." He went on to say that the industry is providing a variety of foods allowing for freedom of choice, that media have sensationalized the results of the randomized trial and misquoted the proper application of these findings, and that the findings apply only to the top 5% of men in whom cholesterol was high. He was, of course, literally correct with regard to the applicability of the findings to the top 5% of men in whom the cholesterol was high. (The National Heart, Lung, and Blood Institute *believes* that the findings might apply to men and women with lower cholesterol levels than those that characterized the study subjects.) However, the Department of Agriculture representative on the same show indicated that people now select lean meat, that the consumption of red meat has been going down, and that of poultry has been increasing. The American Heart Association representative said that "meat should be condiment not central to the meal."

At any rate, even before the firm evidence provided by the randomized trial, dietary changes were already occurring. The industry is modifying its food products to contain a lower proportion of saturated fats, and the population is changing its dietary habits toward more healthful diets. With the new evidence now in hand, further changes on the part of the industry as well as the population should occur, perhaps at an accelerated pace.

CONCLUSION

The firm evidence for the impact of detection, treatment, and control of high blood pressure on reducing mortality and morbidity has led to the adoption of a national policy directed toward this condition. Although they cannot be entirely attributed to this policy, favorable health states are observed.

A national policy may be forthcoming in the light of the similarly firm evidence for the beneficial effects of reducing blood cholesterol.

When high blood pressure and cholesterol are significantly reduced in a large segment of the population, the decline in cardiovascular disease mortality observed since 1968 may even be accelerated. The cost-benefit ratio of preventing coronary heart disease through elimination of risk factors should be contrasted with that resulting from lives lost due to the condition and costs of treatment of survivors in decisions of allocating resources.

BIBLIOGRAPHY

Cochrane AL: *Effectiveness and Efficiency—Random Reflections on Health Services.* London, Nuffield Provisional Hospitals Trust, 1972.

Freis ED: Should mild hypertension be tested? *N Engl J Med* 1982; 307(5): 306–309.

Hausman P: *Jack Sprat's Legacy. The Science and Politics of Fat and Cholesterol.* New York, Richard Marek Publishers, 1981.

Helgeland A: Treatment of mild hypertension: A five year controlled drug trial: The Oslo Study. *Am J Med* 1980; 69: 725–732.

Hypertension Detection and Follow-up Program Cooperative Group: Five-year findings of the hypertension detection and follow-up program. I. Reduction in mortality of persons with high blood pressure, including mild hypertension. *JAMA* 1979; 242: 2562–2571.

Joint National Committee on Detection, Evaluation, and Treatment of High Blood Pressure. The 1984 Report of the Joint National Committee on Detection, Evaluation, and Treatment of High Blood Pressure. *Arch Intern Med* 1984; 144: 1045–1057.

Keys A (ed.): Coronary heart disease in seven countries. *Circulation* 1970; 41: Supplement 1.

Levy RL: The findings of the Hypertension, Detection and Follow-up Program—A multi-year clinical trial. Statement made to the press, Bethesda, Md., 27 November 1979.

Lipid Research Clinics Program: The Lipid Research Clinics Coronary Primary Prevention Trial Results. I. Reduction in incidence of coronary heart disease. *JAMA* 1984; 251: 351–364.

Lipid Research Clinics Program: The Lipid Research Clinics Coronary Primary Prevention Trial Results. II. The relationship of reduction in incidence of coronary heart disease to cholesterol lowering. *JAMA* 1984; 251: 365–374.

Management Committee of the Australian Hypertension Trial: The Australian Therapeutic Trial in Mild Hypertension. *Lancet* 1980; 1: 1261–1269.

Smith WMc: United States Public Health Service Hospitals Cooperative Study Group. Treatment of mild hypertension: Results of a ten-year intervention trial. *Circ Res* 1977, Supplement I, 40(5): 98–105.

Veterans Administration Cooperative Study Group on Antihypertensive Agents: Effects of treatment on morbidity and hypertension. II. Results in patients with diastolic blood pressure averaging 90 through 114 mm Hg. *JAMA* 1970; 213: 1143–1152.

Part VI

Health Care for Selected Populations

Chapter 14

Mothers and Children

Infant and maternal mortality rates are useful indicators not only of the health state of these respective groups but also of the health and socioeconomic levels of a society generally as well as the overall quality of life enjoyed by its citizens. These measures could show large differences over time, between sexes and races, among geographic areas of a country, and among countries.

Infant mortality rates per 1,000 live births have declined over the years. From 1970 to 1980, declines of 38.2% in whites and 34.4% in blacks were noted (Table 14–1). Deaths among infants less than 28 days old, generally reflecting the impact of advanced medical care, have declined 45.7% in whites and 38.2% in blacks. On the other hand deaths among infants 28 days to one year old, generally related to socioeconomic improvements, declined 12.5% in whites but by more than twice that much (26.3%) in blacks.

Maternal mortality—that is, mother's death associated with delivery—has also declined steadily over the years. Like the infant mortality rate, the maternal mortality rate among blacks has been much greater than among whites, and the difference continues in spite of decline of the rate in both groups. Mothers younger than 18 years of age comprise a specific high-risk group. Neonatal mortality rates and postneonatal mortality rates are higher among infants of mothers 17 years of age and younger and multiparas mothers 18 to 19 years of age (McCormick, Shapiro, and Starfield, 1984). A higher proportion of low birth weight infants among this group explains only a portion of the higher mortality rates. The socioeconomic disadvantages of young mothers is another important factor in explaining the higher mortality rates, especially those of the postneonatal period. These findings bear added significance in the light of limited resources available to young mothers and their families to cope with the circumstances arising from

Table 14–1 Infant Mortality Rates per 1,000 Live Births in Whites and Blacks: United States, 1970 and 1980

	Total	< 28 days	28 days–1 year
White			
1970	17.8	13.8	4.0
1980	11.0	7.5	3.5
Percentage of change	−38.2	−45.7	−12.5
Black			
1970	32.6	22.8	9.9
1980	21.4	14.1	7.3
Percentage of change	−34.4	−38.2	−26.3

Source: Adapted from Table 11, National Center for Health Statistics, *Health, United States, 1983,* U.S. Department of Health and Human Services publication no. (PHS) 84–1232 (Washington, D.C.: U.S. Government Printing Office, December 1983), p. 100.

pregnancy and its consequences. The findings of these and other studies provide some rationale for the regionalization of perinatal services, which are discussed later.

Remaining years of life expected at birth and at age 65 have shown a steady increase over the years (Table 14–2). Remaining years expected at birth have increased in the period from 1970 to 1980 by a higher percentage among blacks (6.2% for men and 5.9% for women) than among whites (4.0% for men and 3.3% for women). At age 65, the opposite trend was noted: white men gained 8.4% but black men gained 3.2%, and white women gained 8.2% but black women gained 5.1%.

Infant mortality rates and life expectancies also vary in different countries (Table 14–3). Sweden and Japan top the list with the lowest infant mortality rates and the highest life expectancies. In Canada, England and Wales, and the United States, infant mortality rates and life expectancies are similar.

The declines in infant and maternal mortalities have been due largely to improvements in socioeconomic conditions as well as in the quality of medical care. Regular and timely prenatal care of good quality is one of the most important preventive measures for pregnant women. The first trimester is the best time for the initiation of prenatal care. There has been a gradual increase in the proportion of white and black women who began prenatal care in the first trimester of pregnancy. An increase of 11% from 72% to 80% between the years of 1970 and

Table 14–2 Remaining Life Expectancy in Years at Birth and at 65 Years of Age by Race and Sex, United States, 1970 and 1980

	White Men	White Women	Black Men	Black Women
At Birth				
1970	68.0	75.6	60.0	68.3
1980	70.7	78.1	63.7	72.3
Percentage of change	+ 4.0	+ 3.3	+ 6.2	+ 5.9
At Age 65				
1970	13.1	17.1	12.5	15.7
1980	14.2	18.5	12.9	16.5
Percentage of change	+ 8.4	+ 8.2	+ 3.2	+ 5.1

Source: Adapted from Table 10, National Center for Health Statistics, *Health, United States, 1983,* U.S. Department of Health and Human Services publication no. (PHS) 84–1232 (Washington, D.C.: U.S. Government Printing Office, December 1983), p. 99.

Table 14–3 Infant Mortality Rates per 1,000 Live Births and Life Expectancy at Birth, Selected Countries, 1976–1980

	Infant Mortality	Life Expectancy Men	Life Expectancy Women
Sweden	6.7	72.5	78.7
Japan	7.4	73.5	78.9
France	9.9	69.9	78.0
Australia	11.0	70.8	77.8
Canada	11.9	70.2	77.5
England & Wales	11.9	70.0	76.2
United States	12.6	69.9	77.6
German Federal Republic	13.5	69.0	75.6
Greece	18.7	70.8	75.0

Source: Adapted from Tables 13 and 14, National Center for Health Statistics, *Health, United States, 1983,* U.S. Department of Health and Human Services publication no. (PHS) 84–1232 (Washington, D.C.: U.S. Government Printing Office, December 1983), pp. 103–104.

1980, respectively, has occurred among white women. The comparable increase among black women was 33%, from 45% to about 60% (National Center for Health Statistics, December 1983). In spite of these gains, 20% of white women, and 40% of black women, did not begin their prenatal care at the proper time, that is, in the first trimester.

EPIDEMIOLOGIC ANALYSIS OF EXISTING DATA

Reducing maternal and infant deaths remains an important objective for the nation. In 1933 a report entitled *Maternal Mortality in New York City. A Study of All Puerperal Deaths 1930–1932* was published (New York Academy of Medicine Committee on Public Health Relations, 1933). Examination of autopsy findings, interviews with physicians, and an assessment of preventability were carefully made in every maternal death. The maternal mortality in New York City, about 57 per 10,000 live births, was considered very high, especially in the light of the conclusion of the New York Academy of Medicine that about two-thirds of the deaths could have been prevented.

The academy report was perhaps of special significance as were the reports on mental retardation commissioned by President Kennedy in the early 1960s and the report on heart disease, cancer, and stroke commissioned by President Johnson in the late 1960s. The report on maternal deaths "was enormously successful in introducing needed reforms which contributed to the dramatic decline in maternal deaths over the subsequent decades" (Schaffner et al. 1977, p. 821). Similar committees were formed in many states including Michigan, where epidemiologic analysis of available data provided important information for action.

Data for 22 years (1950–71) were compiled on the causes of maternal deaths and their correlates (Schaffner et al. 1977). Over that period, the maternal death rate declined from 5 per 10,000 births in 1960 to 1.5 in 1971. Although the rates for whites and blacks declined considerably, the maternal death rate among blacks continued to be much greater than that for whites (Figure 14–1).

The relationship between maternal deaths and maternal age was portrayed in a typical J curve (Figure 14–1). The rate was high in those younger than 15 years of age but highest in those 40 years of age and older. Continuous rise was noted from a lowest rate in those 15 to 19 years of age to higher rates in the older age groups. Blacks experienced higher maternal death rates than whites at every maternal age group.

The relationship between maternal deaths and parity was confounded by maternal age (Figure 14–1). Without adjustment for age, the crude death rate increased gradually as the number of previous live births increased but showed a steep rise in mothers with seven or more previous live births. This trend, however, disappeared after adjustment for age, indicating that the relationship to parity is a function of increased age of the mother rather than increased number of previous live births.

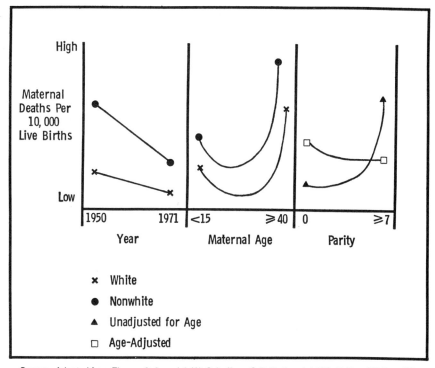

Source: Adapted from Figures 2, 3, and 4, W. Schaffner, C.F. Federspiel, M.L. Fulton, "Maternal Mortality in Michigan: An Epidemiologic Analysis, 1950–1971," *American Journal of Public Health* 1977 (67): 821–829.

Figure 14–1 Schematic Representation of Maternal Deaths over Time and Relationships to Maternal Age and Parity

Although the relationship between maternal deaths and parity was clarified by adjusting for mother's age, it is important to note the different implications of this observation for etiologic and health service research. Age was a confounding factor that explained the relationship between maternal deaths and maternal age—an important observation in research aimed at the elucidation of causal factors. However, women with increased numbers of previous live births do experience higher maternal mortality rates—an important fact to bear in mind when planning for services for such women in spite of the fact that their increased risk to maternal deaths is generally due to their older age.

A final and important finding of the study in terms of health policy was the relationship between maternal deaths and the size of the obstetrical service. Maternal deaths were found inversely related to the size of the obstetrical unit in a given hospital. The rate in hospitals with less than 4 live births per week was more than six times the rate in hospitals with 85 or more live births per week.

Preventable deaths were estimated at 71% during the period of study, with an increase from a rate of 58% in 1950 to about 85% in 1971. Hemorrhage was the leading cause of death among whites and of infection among blacks. Preventable deaths were generally higher in rural areas than in urban areas and among blacks than among whites.

The pattern of maternal deaths over time, relationships to maternal age, parity, and size of obstetrical service as well as the proportion that is preventable provide important information for policy development. Targeting services to the group at highest risk and most vulnerable is one approach. Another might be found in the regionalization of perinatal services, which would allow sharing of sophisticated services, targeting appropriate services to appropriate groups at risk, and transmitting and applying new information rapidly.

IMPACT OF MATERNAL MORTALITY STUDY COMMITTEES

The role of state maternal mortality study committees in the decline of maternal mortality rates over time has not been clear. Rates of decline from 1940 to 1970 were compared for states with committees to those without (Grimes and Cates 1977). Maternal deaths and live births for each state of residence were obtained from published vital statistics, and the dates of establishing maternal mortality study committees were obtained from the results of a survey (Grimes and Cates 1977). States with and states without committees experienced more or less the same decline in maternal mortality rates, and there was no essential difference between them. Committees might have had an impact, but it was probably confounded by coincidental and dramatic improvements in health care, which led to reductions in maternal and infant mortalities.

What did such committees actually do? The formation of these committees represents measures of services, processes, or effort. The changes desired might have been the education of physicians; prenatal care delivered to more pregnant women, especially those at high risk; and investigation of maternal deaths to inquire about possible preventable causes. These are the changes that would ultimately result in the decreased maternal mortality.

Unfortunately inferences cannot be readily made about the potential impact of such committees. If there were no relationship as has been shown earlier, the role of confounding factors cannot be easily ruled out. If on the other hand there were an association between committee initiation and decreased maternal mortality, the simple comparison of states with and states without would not necessarily answer the question. Confounding factors might have been responsible for the changes in the states with committees. Randomization of maternal mortality study committees to states or locales and measurement of end results would have provided firm evidence as to the impact of such committees.

HOME CARE

Midwifery and home deliveries were popular at the turn of the century when about half of all deliveries were performed by midwives (Williams 1912). This peak in midwifery and home deliveries began to decline in 1936, when midwives accounted for 12% of all deliveries, and by 1952 accounted for only 4½% (Hunt and Moore 1958). After further decline in the 1950s and 1960s, midwifery and home delivery began to rise again. However, home deliveries make only about 1% of all deliveries (National Center for Health Statistics, 1982). Those who opt for home deliveries are generally women of the upper and middle social classes. Hospitals are responding by providing what is called *birth centers,* where "humane" treatment and comfortable "nonhospital" environment are provided. The extent to which the home delivery movement will grow is unknown.

The rise and fall of the popularity of home deliveries coincides with the increased or decreased interest in midwifery. In 1978 the Arizona Department of Health Services adopted rules and regulations to ensure adequate quality of care as part of the process of licensing midwives in that state (Sullivan and Beeman 1983). Maternal and newborn outcomes were evaluated during a four-year period between 1978 and 1981, when 26 licensed midwives delivered 1,243 babies, or less than 1% of Arizona's total live births. About 3% of mothers were hospitalized for complications, and 5% of the babies required medical attention. The proportion of women with a shorter length of labor and less blood loss during labor has increased over the years. Complications requiring postmortem attention decreased from 29% in 1978 to 16% in 1981, a reduction of 45%. These data suggest that "home births can be a safe alternative for low-risk pregnancies" provided proper safeguards are taken (Sullivan and Beeman 1983, p. 645).

The increased interest in home deliveries has rekindled questions regarding the effectiveness of home services generally. Health assessments and counseling of women before and after delivery at home by public health nurses have been provided for years—services that "still comprise the major portion of the overall nursing program in many official health agencies" (Barkauskas 1983, p. 573). The impact of public health nursing services on the health of mothers and infants seems to be insignificant (Barkauskas 1983). Home services generally and home services by public health nurses need to be reexamined insofar as benefits and costs are concerned.

SPECIFIC HEALTH PROBLEMS AND BEHAVIORS

Selected health problems associated with motherhood and women generally have been the subject of many surveys. The rising Caesarean section delivery rate in the United States is noteworthy (Placek, Taffel, and Moien 1983). The rate increased from 4.5 per 100 deliveries in 1965 to about 18 per 100 deliveries in 1981. The highest rates were noted in hospitals of 500 beds or more, in proprietary hospitals, and when Blue Cross was the source of payment (Placek, Taffel, and Moien 1983). Incidence of ectopic pregnancies in women aged 15–55 also witnessed a rise from 56 to 84 per 100,000 women from 1972 to 1978 (Shiono, Harlap, and Pellegrin 1982). Methods of birth control and changes in birth control practices may have been playing a part in the rising incidence of ectopic pregnancies, which has occurred mostly in women 30 years old and younger. Hysterectomies in women 15 years old and older are performed at a rate of 4.4 per 1,000 women in Manitoba and 6.7 in the United States (Roos 1984).

The benefits and risks associated with hysterectomy are matters of considerable concern. Although the mortality from the operation itself is low, there is an increased number of complications requiring hospitalization, as well as more visits to physicians as a result of psychological, urinary tract infection, and menopausal problems. The rise in these conditions and the associated morbidity and mortality require closer monitoring to aid in the proper allocation of resources.

Periodic breast self-examination and mammography are important preventive services for breast cancer. The practice of breast self-examination several times annually was not associated with significant results in comparison to monthly practice (Feldman et al. 1981). Furthermore, regular practice was associated with reduced likelihood of the diagnosis of breast cancer with involvement of the lymph nodes, which "translated to a 10% decline in five-year mortality for whites and a 17% decline for non-whites" (Feldman et al. 1981, p. 2740). Knowledge about mammography and attitudes about it were described in a representative sample of women living in Los Angeles (Berkanovic and Reeder 1979). A large proportion of women (40%) have not heard of the procedure, but only 11% of those who had heard about it expressed negative feelings.

These observations and the associated morbidity, mortality, and costs require close monitoring. They should be considered in allocating resources. Regionalization of perinatal care as described next is one example.

REGIONALIZATION OF PERINATAL CARE

Given that the distribution of perinatal services, especially those requiring sophisticated and expensive devices or procedures, is uneven, and that morbidity and mortality of mothers and infants are higher in certain areas and groups than others, the concept of regionalization may provide a good alternative for both scientific and economic reasons. Regionalization of perinatal care would involve defined geographic areas and population groups, especially the high-risk groups, and would require the sharing of resources and services, which ultimately should result in efficiency, cost saving, and better health states of the population served.

The impetus for regionalization stems from the rapid development of sophisticated procedures such as ultrasound and fetal monitoring, which are widely used in many medical care facilities. Allocation of resources on the basis of a regionalization concept should ideally be accompanied by proper evaluation of its worth in order that appropriate policies may be formulated in this regard.

A pilot project "in a five-county underserved, predominantly rural area with a high average perinatal mortality (1973–1975) rate of 31.5 per 1,000" was launched in North Carolina as a model project for devising an evaluation of such endeavors (Siegel et al. 1977, p. 286). These counties presented an ideal opportunity for a regionalized program since they were predominantly rural, with high perinatal mortality and morbidity, and probably in need of sophisticated perinatal care. The project was implemented after the North Carolina legislature passed a perinatal health care bill in 1974 and appropriated $500,000, which in addition to $750,000 from the federal government was sufficient to begin a regionalized program.

The *services* to be provided included establishing perinatal clinics for high-risk mothers, forming consultative and referral networks with the teaching medical centers in North Carolina, linking existing as well as new services in a coordinated system, and developing service statistics for visit frequencies and referrals (Siegel et al. 1977).

An elaborate and complete information system was essential for determining the impact on health states of such reorganization. Needed information was collected on perinatal and postpartum visits and family planning visits to health departments, but "efforts to collect the same information on an ongoing basis in private physicians' offices failed," which required that information on samples of private physicians be collected retrospectively (Siegel et al. 1977, p. 290).

The *outcome indicators* were carefully outlined before the implementation of the program (Siegel et al. 1977). These included reduction in the percentage of high-risk births, such as those occurring to mothers younger than 18 years of age or with less than 9 years of education, and of unwanted births. Other indicators included reduction in the percentage of women with an unfavorable pregnancy course, such as those developing blood pressure greater than 140/90 at delivery, reduction in perinatal morbidity and mortality, and reduction in long-term perinatal morbidity.

With the services outlined as well as the outcomes of such services, the *changes* must also be documented, as described in Chapter 1. The changes in this case would mean achievement of the following endeavors such as

90% of all pregnant women receive the first prenatal visit before the 16th week of pregnancy . . . 90% of all pregnant women receive five or more prenatal visits . . . 95% of all high-risk mothers and infants receive consultation . . . 90% of all high-risk mothers and infants are treated in the center most appropriate to their needs . . . review (of) all cases of perinatal mortality. (Siegel et al. 1977, p. 295)

An outcome variable such as perinatal death rates over time in the program area in contrast to the comparison area may be used as an illustration of program impact. As schematically represented in Figure 14–2, the comparison area was experiencing a similar decline in perinatal mortality death rate as was the program area, which was important to note so as not to credit the program unduly. However, after regionalization was implemented in 1975, it might be expected that the rate of decline of perinatal deaths among the program area residents would be faster than that among the residents of the comparison area. If similar findings were shown in other end results, which could be linked effectively to the expected

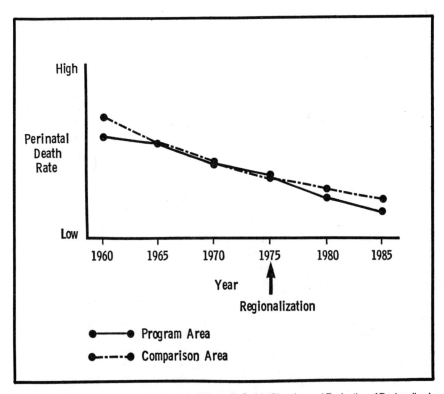

Source: Adapted from Table 5, E. Siegel, D. Gillings, P. Guild, "Planning and Evaluation of Regionalized Perinatal Care: A Rural Example," *Seminars in Perinatology* 1977 1(3): 283–301.

Figure 14–2 Schematic Representation of Impact of Regionalization on Perinatal Mortality

changes, and if the improvement in outcome could be related in a dose-response relationship in that better outcomes are achieved when the amount of service is increased, then the evidence for beneficial effects of regionalization may be considered persuasive.

CONCLUSION

Mother and infant health indicators have been important parameters of gauging the health state and socioeconomic development of areas and countries. Epidemiologic information is generally available from birth certificates, vital statistics, and records of physicians and hospitals. These data provide important resources of information for examining health states of populations, planning and evaluating various programs including regionalization, and aiding in policy decisions with regard to allocation of costly or sophisticated procedures and devices.

Regionalization of perinatal care services need not be limited to this type of medical practice. Indeed there was some interest in the mid-1960s through the resources of the Regional Medical Programs introduced in President Johnson's administration to regionalize medical services, especially those for coronary heart disease and stroke. In addition to other attempts to control costs and democratize accessibility to medical care, regionalization may be a concept worthy of serious consideration.

BIBLIOGRAPHY

Barkauskas VH: Effectiveness of public health nurse home visits to primarous mothers and their infants. *Am J Public Health* 1983; 73: 573–580.

Berkanovic E, Reeder SJ: Awareness, opinion, and behavioral intention of urban women regarding mammography. *Am J Public Health* 1979; 69: 1172–1174.

Feldman JG, Carter AC, Nicastri AD et al: Breast self-examination, relationship to stage of breast cancer at diagnosis. *Cancer* 1981; 47: 2740–2745.

Grimes DA, Cates W Jr: The impact of state maternal mortality study committees on natural deaths in the United States. *Am J Public Health* 1977; 67: 830–833.

Hunt EP, Moore RR: *Perinatal, Infant, Childhood, and Maternal Mortality,* Children's Bureau Statistical Series No. 50. Washington, DC, Social Security Administration, Children's Bureau, 1958. Cited in Yankauer A: The valley of the shadow of birth, editorial. *Am J Public Health* 1983, 73(6): 635–638.

McCormick MC, Shapiro S, Starfield B: High-risk young mothers: Infant mortality and morbidity in four areas in the United States, 1973–1978. *Am J Public Health* 1984; 74: 18–23.

National Center for Health Statistics: *Advance Report of Final Natality Statistics, 1980.* Monthly Vital Statistics Report 31, No. 8, suppl. Washington, DC, US Dept of Health and Human Services, November 30, 1982. Cited in Yankauer A: The valley of the shadow of birth, editorial. *Am J Public Health* 1983, 73(6): 635–638.

National Center for Health Statistics: *Health, United States, 1982*, US Dept of Health and Human Services Publication No. (PHS) 83–1232. Government Printing Office, December 1982.

National Center for Health Statistics: *Health, United States, 1983*, US Dept of Health and Human Services Publication No. (PHS) 84–1232. Government Printing Office, December 1983.

New York Academy of Medicine Committee on Public Health Relations: *Maternal Mortality in New York City. A Study of All Puerperal Deaths 1930–32*. New York, The Commonwealth Fund, Oxford University Press, 1933. Cited in Schaffner W et al: Maternal mortality in Michigan: An epidemiologic analysis, 1950–1971. *Am J Public Health* 1977; 67: 821–829.

Placek PJ, Taffel S, Moien M: Cesarean section delivery rates: United States, 1981. *Am J Public Health* 1983; 73: 861–862.

Roos NP: Hysterectomies in one Canadian province: A new look at risks and benefits. *Am J Public Health* 1984; 74: 39–46.

Schaffner W, Federspiel CF, Fulton ML et al: Maternal mortality in Michigan: An epidemiologic analysis, 1950–1971. *Am J Public Health* 1977; 67: 821–829.

Shiono PH, Harlap S, Pellegrin F: Ectopic pregnancies: Rising incidence rates in northern California. *Am J Public Health* 1982; 72: 173–175.

Siegel E, Gillings D, Guild P et al: Planning and evaluation of regionalized perinatal care: A rural example. *Seminars in Perinatology* 1977; 1(3): 283–301.

Sullivan DA, Beeman R: Four years' experience with home birth by licensed midwives in Arizona. *Am J Public Health* 1983; 73: 641–645.

Williams JW: Medical education and the midwife problem in the United States. *JAMA* 1912; 58: 1–7. Cited in Yankauer A: The valley of the shadow of birth, editorial. *Am J Public Health* 1983, 73 (6): 635–638.

Chapter 15

The Aged

Can an affluent society afford to meet predictably increasing health care costs for an inevitably increasing elderly population and meet the added costs of new programs of health promotion and maintenance?

Amasa B. Ford

The elderly segment is increasing both in terms of the proportion of the entire population and in absolute numbers. In 1980, 25 million individuals were 65 years of age and older and accounted for 11 percent of the population. Because of differential mortality between the sexes, women outnumber men by a ratio of 10 to 7. Heart disease, cancer, and stroke are the leading causes of death. Chronic disabilities, dependence, loneliness, poor housing, and relative inaccessibility of medical care because of geography or cost compound the problem of the aged.

The most widely publicized health care policy issue is that of cost and cost containment since the elderly utilize resources at a much higher rate than their proportion of the population. One of the most important questions is where an individual should be looked after: day care center, senior citizen center, own home, nursing home, or hospital. The placement question is important not only for patient and family consideration but also for cost. Sophisticated technologies—diagnostic, therapeutic, and rehabilitative—continue to emerge, and their use in hospitals and similar facilities for an expanding elderly population with enormous chronic problems will certainly contribute to rising costs.

The most significant health care policy issue is that concerning the various facets of providing long-term care for the elderly. This issue is addressed first and is followed by methods of measurement of health and functional states of the elderly. Viewed as end results, health and functional status should provide important clues for deciding on the most appropriate mode for long-term care. Finally, two different views on aging, one of which highlights the potential impact of health promotion, are summarized. These views, which introduce fresh ideas, help focus our thinking on what the future for the aged population might look like.

LONG-TERM CARE

Long-term care represents a crucial aspect of needed services for the elderly. Since life expectancies and prevalence of chronic illnesses are expected to continue their trends, more elderly people and more chronic conditions would require long-term care including institutionalization. The proper placement of the elderly depends on the degree of disability and available community and family resources. It also depends on incentives or disincentives of the Medicare and Medicaid reimbursement policies. It is important to note that "institutionalization in nursing homes is common for the approximately 5 percent of elderly who need constant personal care. The alternatives to institutionalization (such as home health care, day health care, and organized ambulatory care) are largely experimental at present" (Pegels 1980, 134).

Long-term care may be examined from a financial aspect as well as from an epidemiologic vantage point making use of the findings of comparative studies. The system of financing long-term care, whether through Medicare or Medicaid, seems inadequate as it separates the financing of care for the chronically ill and disabled from the financing of acute care (Somers 1982). Support for a separate long-term care system comes from two opposing groups; one believes that keeping it separate would give it sufficient prominence and keep it out of the domination of physicians, and another group who actually supports the acute care system would like to keep long-term care separate so that it will not "seriously dilute the funds now available for acute care" (Somers 1982, p. 223). At any rate, integration of long-term care with acute care may be the subject of further study.

The scientific base with regard to the impact of available options on health states and to the costs of these options remains meager. An enlightened policy on this matter would benefit from scientific information. Alternatives to institutionalization in long-term care plans are attractive not only because of cost savings but for the provision of a more comfortable environment for the elderly. Home-based care, which is generally provided by family members, is one of the options. About 2 per 100 elderly per year enter a long-term care institution. What are the characteristics of these individuals? Targeting specific services to the elderly may take advantage of the fact that "advancing age, using ambulatory aids, mental disorientation, living alone, and using assistance to perform 'instrumental' ADL (activities of daily living)" are associated with institutionalization (Branch and

Jette 1982, p. 1373). These variables explain only about 10% of the variance of long-term-care institutionalization. Other unknown factors are yet to be discovered through further research.

Institutional care policies would have benefited from good research before "its foundations were laid down in the Social Security Act which brought into being our present system of (mainly proprietary) nursing home" (Morris 1980, p. 471). This system, coupled with the lack of criteria for "slotting people into at-home or institutional care," resulted in practices which are "reflexive and *ad hoc*" (Morris 1980, p. 472). What is needed is better methods of assessing impairments in the elderly so that proper placements can be made. More studies on the various options and their impact on the health of the elderly may provide a better basis for policy formulation than is currently available.

MEASUREMENT OF HEALTH STATE

One of the most widely used measurements of health state in the elderly is the Index of Activity of Daily Living (ADL) (Katz et al. 1970). The index quantifies functions of bathing, dressing, going to toilet, transferring, continence, and feeding. For each of these functions, responses to questions are categorized into those requiring no assistance, some assistance, or a lot of assistance. Functional capacity is graded from A to G, indicating a continuum from the most dependent to the most independent. The scale has been validated in several studies in which increasing dependence according to the index was found to be associated with increasing proportion of individuals who were found in nursing homes, hospitals, or custodial institutions (Katz et al. 1970).

The index may be used for predicting assistance needs to aid clinicians in choosing a therapeutic course. In examining the option of care services for the elderly, the index is useful for a prerandomization stratification analysis of the study population to enhance representation of all levels of functioning. The index may also be used as an outcome variable to gauge the impact of services on the functional status of the patient. It could be further used in postrandomization stratification analysis to examine various outcome variables in specific functional classes.

The Activity of Daily Living Index, which was also referred to in Chapter 2, is therefore an important instrument in health service research for the elderly population. The general question of measurement and classification of health states in the elderly must be considered with reference to an emerging trend of two groups of people 65 years and older. These are "the junior elderly consisting of those from 65–75, and the senior elderly consisting of those 75 and over" (Pegels 1980, p. 212). These would seem to be two distinct groups with different functional status and health care needs. Further research on these issues is in order.

CONCEPTUAL VIEWS ABOUT AGING

The aged population is increasing both in absolute numbers and in the proportion of the population at large; it suffers from a high prevalence of chronic diseases. The recent declines in mortality, especially due to cardiovascular and cerebrovascular diseases, affected those 85 years of age and older. The decline of mortality in the elderly coupled with prevalent chronic conditions and poor health might result in a large number of elderly people who are suffering from chronic conditions and disabilities and, therefore, a "burgeoning number of patients in need of long-term care" (Schneider and Brody 1983, p. 855).

If it is assumed on the other hand that the length of human life is fixed and that preventive measures could successfully postpone the onset of chronic conditions in the aged population, then it may be predicted that the number of very old people would not increase in the years ahead and that chronic diseases would occur in a smaller proportion of the aged, thus resulting in a decrease in medical care services needed by the elderly (Fries 1980).

The projected fixed length of life is based on the assumption that the deterioration of organ functions with increasing age is associated with exponential increase in mortality after age 30, and together should result in a fixed life span. Since life expectancy has hardly increased for those 75 years of age and older, and as premature deaths are reduced, the progressive "rectangularization" of the survival curve would occur. Changes in life style and better treatment may have contributed to the decline in premature deaths and may contribute to "compression" of morbidity "into the shorter span between the increasing age at onset of disability and the fixed occurrence of death . . . thus results in rectangularization not only of the mortality curve but also of the morbidity curve" (Fries 1980, p. 133).

If these predictions were upheld,

> the number of very old persons will not increase . . . the average period of diminished physical vigor will decrease . . . chronic disease will occupy a smaller proportion of the typical life span . . . the time between birth and first permanent infirmity must increase . . . the average period of infirmity must decrease . . . the need for medical care in later life will decrease. (Fries 1980, p. 130)

These predictions—as attractive as they may appear—can be challenged on the basis of current facts and trends. A different conclusion could be reached in that the number of very old people will increase, the period of diminished vigor will increase, and chronic diseases will occur in a large proportion of the elderly, and all that will result in increased demand for medical care. This position has been outlined so that "Fries' seductive predictions will not be used for health-care planning and policy decisions, and that valuable resources will not be diverted from programs directed at the prevention and treatment of chronic diseases'' (Schneider and Brody 1983, p. 855).

Health promotion and disease prevention efforts should be viewed beyond the arguments of medical care resources and costs. The impact of such measures requires lead time before benefits could be adequately demonstrated. Conditions revealed by screening procedures, for example, would require medical attention with its concomitant costs. When certain conditions in the elderly are eliminated or postponed, other conditions may take their place. Furthermore, several intervention activities have yet to be shown to result in perceptible changes in health states.

CONCLUSION

''The marked increase in the number of very old individuals is the reward for better housing, improved sanitation, efficient medical and nursing services. These new years of life must be regarded as a prize, and society must be prepared to provide the amount of help required by senior citizens to keep them healthy'' (Anderson 1982, p. 109). A national health policy, coherent and coordinated, for the elderly is overdue.

BIBLIOGRAPHY

Anderson WF: Is health education for middle-aged and elderly a waste of time? in Wells T (ed.): *Aging and Health Promotion*. Rockville, Md, Aspen Systems Corp, 1982.

Branch LG, Jette AM: A prospective study of long-term care institutionalization among the aged. *Am J Public Health* 1982; 72(12): 1373–1379.

Ford AB: Is health promotion affordable for the elderly? in Wells T (ed.): *Aging and Health Promotion*. Rockville, Md, Aspen Systems Corp, 1982.

Fries JF: Aging, natural death, and the compression of morbidity. *N Engl Med* 1980; 303(3): 130–135.

Katz S, Downs TD, Cash HR et al: Progress in development of the index of ADL. *Gerontologist* 1970; 10(1): 20–30.

Morris R: Designing care for the long-term patient: How much change is necessary in the pattern of health provision? editorial. *Am J Public Health* 1980; 70(5): 471–472.

Pegels CC: *Health Care and the Elderly*. Rockville, Md, Aspen Systems Corp, 1980.

Schneider EL, Brody JA: Aging, natural death, and the compression of morbidity: Another view. *N Engl J Med* 1983; 309(14): 854–856.

Somers AR: Long-term care for the elderly and disabled. A new health priority. *N Engl J Med* 1982; 307(4): 221–226.

Epilogue

Numerous questions were raised and some were answered in this text. All are pivotal in setting policy for health care. As important as they are, political and economic concerns must not be the sole determinants of policy. Epidemiologic and other scientific evidence that is focused on the impact of a health program or procedure on health states of populations must be seriously taken into account in making policy.

Are there situations in which neither health policy nor rigorous scientific evidence exist? Technologies have spread widely without policy and before scientific evidence of benefits has accrued. The use and acceptance of intensive care units, computed tomography, and coronary bypass surgery made scientific evidence more difficult to accumulate.

Do situations exist in which there is health policy without scientific evidence? In fact there are only a few situations in which there is any sort of policy. Nevertheless a national policy was advanced when a campaign to immunize the American population in 1975 against swine flu was mounted before all available evidence was considered carefully. The policy was halted shortly after it was initiated because of complications from the vaccine and negative public reaction to the whole idea.

Do situations exist in which there is no policy but there is reliable scientific evidence? New health professionals whose practices have been proven safe and efficacious continue to participate in the health care system without a clear policy defining their place in the system.

Do situations exist in which there are both policy and evidence? A case in point is the establishment of comprehensive national programs to control high blood pressure after randomized trials had produced conclusive results.

Scientific evidence must inevitably play a key role in the formulation of health policies. Examples of policy founded on such evidence are becoming more abundant. A national policy to reduce high blood cholesterol, would seem logical, based on persuasive supporting evidence that mortality would be reduced as a result. Epidemiology as a factor in health policy is an idea whose time has come.

Index

About the Author

Michel A. Ibrahim was trained in medicine at the University of Cairo (MD, 1957) and in biostatistics (MPH, 1961) and epidemiology (PhD, 1964) at the University of North Carolina School of Public Health. He is currently dean and professor of epidemiology in that school and was chairman of its department of epidemiology from 1976 to 1982. Previous positions in Buffalo were Deputy Health Commissioner of Erie County, and Associate Professor at the University of New York School of Medicine.

Dr. Ibrahim is a member of several scientific journal editorial boards, National Institutes of Health advisory groups, and policy boards concerned with environment, cancer, heart disease, and medical care. He is a fellow of the American Public Health Association, the American Heart Association, and the American College of Epidemiology.

Dr. Ibrahim has conducted and published research on the epidemiology and medical care of cardiovascular diseases, the evaluation of primary medical care, the assessment of clinical skills of health care practitioners, the application of epidemiology to health services, the case-control study designs, and the incorporation of hypertension control programs in rural communities.